TEACH YOURSELF

Yoga

26/10/21

TEACH YOURSELF

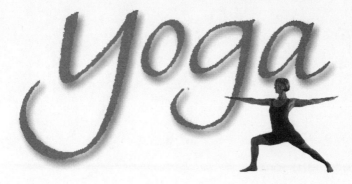

Yoga

EVE GRZYBOWSKI

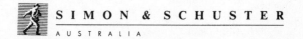

SIMON & SCHUSTER
AUSTRALIA

TEACH YOURSELF YOGA

First published in Australasia in 1997 by
Simon & Schuster Australia
20 Barcoo Street, East Roseville NSW 2069

A Viacom Company
Sydney New York London Toronto Tokyo Singapore

© Eve Grzybowski 1997

National Library of Australia
Cataloguing-in-Publication data

Grzybowski, Eve
    Teach yourself yoga.

    Bibliography.
    ISBN 0 7318 0640 9.

    1. Yoga. 2. Yoga, Hatha. 3. Astanga yoga. I. Title.

613.7046

Design by Anna Soo
Photography by David Clare
Printed in Australia by Griffin Press

To my teachers for the gift of my passion for yoga
And to my students for keeping the fire kindled.

FOREWORD

When I discovered yoga, my life changed. The changes have been slow and subtle, but nevertheless profound. From my very first yoga class, I knew it was for me. I remember coming out of the class feeling like I was walking on air with my head in the clouds! Gradually, over time, I started to feel more comfortable with, and in, my body. The niggly aches and pains I used to feel have been replaced by a sense of wellbeing and my muscles are more relaxed, stronger and more flexible.

Eve became one of my favourite teachers. Watching her demonstrate a yoga pose with superb grace is like watching a moving piece of art. You know you won't be able to reproduce it exactly, but with her gentle encouragement and faith in your ability you quite often surprise yourself.

The big turning point in my life came when Eve suggested I sign up for the yoga teaching training course. I had secretly dreamed of doing it, but convinced myself I wasn't quite up to scratch. As soon as I heard those encouraging words, I started to feel more confident about being good enough to take on the course. As it turned out, that year was the best of my life. I loved every minute of the course and learnt a lot about myself — and my yoga improved out of sight.

Life is a journey and yoga has helped me confront that journey head on. It has been like a road map for me, gently giving me directions to the pathways I need to take. Yoga helped me make the inner connection with myself, allowing me to choose the smooth path instead of the rocky road.

It is a great honour for me to recommend Eve's book. I have collected many great yoga books over the years, but this one truly stands out as a gem. Eve's warm and caring nature shines through the pages. Her personable style draws you in immediately, keeping you hungry for more. Covering every aspect of yoga, *Teach Yourself Yoga* is easy to read and understand — so whether you're a complete beginner or someone who's travelled the yoga path for a while, you'll find it equally useful.

Teach Yourself Yoga will become an essential handbook to read and re-read for practical knowledge and inspiration.

Alison King
Products Editor, *Family Circle,* and yoga teacher

CONTENTS

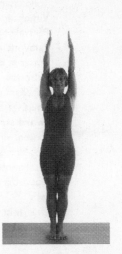

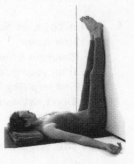

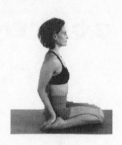

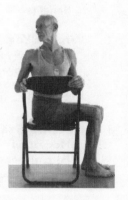

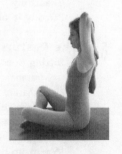

ACKNOWLEDGMENTS

I'm grateful for the clear thinking beginner's mind my husband, Daniel Weinstein, brought to reading the early and later versions of this book; the constructive criticism and friendship of Michael Hollingworth and Heather Hyde; the 'you-can-do-it' attitude of Lynne Segal; the enthusiasm and editing art of Brigitta Doyle; and the willing offers of computer support from my stepson, Ben Weinstein.

INTRODUCTION

The image people have of yoga, a 3000-year-old discipline, has been undergoing rapid, and radical, change. In recent times, it has become popular and 'trendy', even among the celebrity set. It would be fair to say that yoga has finally arrived!

This became obvious to me when, a few months ago, I was contacted by a journalist from a major daily newspaper who wanted to interview me about yoga for a cover story in the paper's weekend magazine. To many yoga teachers and students, the article that appeared wasn't a hot news item. But the story did give credibility to the idea that yoga is an intelligent exercise system, and a great alternative and/or complement to stress sports (such as running, swimming, aerobics) and gym exercise.

Yoga's main advantage is that it works well for *everyone*, regardless of age, occupation, status or level of fitness. People are discovering that yoga serves their physical, emotional, mental and spiritual needs, and that it has more depth and staying power than other exercise systems around.

Of course, I'm biased. Yoga is the longest-lasting relationship I've had — one that's engaged my body, mind and soul for more than 25 years.

I made my yoga debut in the early 1970s. Yoga was then a fairly far-fetched idea, even though it had been around, in one form or another, for a very long time. It was introduced to the West in the late 1700s (through translations of Hindu works of literature), and has since slowly infiltrated our culture.

I didn't know what I was getting myself into when a friend

dragged me along to a 10-week YMCA course. I just thought, 'What the heck'. When the course finished, I lost track of my friend and I don't know if she ever did another yoga class in her life. But for me, the combination of being physically challenged while learning to relax really clicked.

As a child, I was very physical and loved anything athletic. Then, over the years, sport made my body tight and my back weak. When I started attending the YMCA yoga classes, I was faced with loosening up my chronically tight body and working with my weak back. I found it a revelation that yoga's relaxed approach to exercise could make the exercise more effective.

I had to stop attending classes because it was difficult to arrange child care for my son, but I bought a yoga book, made my own stick drawings of the postures on some cards and began to practise on my own. Through daily repetition, I gradually taught myself many of the postures. I never looked back. From the very start, I felt I was getting more out of the practice than I put into it.

My son was about two years old then, and when I put him down for an afternoon nap, that was *my time* — and I used it to do my yoga practice.

I teach many new mothers yoga these days and I understand how absolutely crucial this 'alone-time' is for them. Because of the stresses of family life, it's essential for new mothers to have a regular time for replenishing themselves and turning their attention inwards. (I discuss this further on pages 49–51 and describe a sequence of poses for pre- and postnatal women.)

At the yoga school I founded in Sydney, I was surprised to discover during the last recession that our class attendance soared. People came along not just to gain suppleness and strength, but to unwind and to be reminded how to breathe. It's remarkable that people actually need to learn how to breathe! It shows how far we've strayed from our most natural impulse.

Owing to the stress we face in our daily lives — juggling work commitments, relationships, family and so on — we'd be hard-pressed to find anyone who wasn't battling to cope to some degree. Even the Dalai Lama and the Tibetan monks on their mountain tops in Northern India are working hard every day to free Tibet! Stress is here to stay, so we need to find coping mechanisms.

When I started yoga, the selection of easy-to-understand yoga books was limited and the explanation of postures was not easy to grasp. It is my intention in *Teach Yourself Yoga* to present a simple and interesting introduction to yoga, so that you will feel motivated to practise *and* enjoy it.

Teach Yourself Yoga is designed to benefit you on all levels — mind, body and spirit. I hope to inspire you through examples of my own experiences and the experiences of other yoga practitioners (yogis).

In describing the yoga poses and yoga philosophy, I've used Sanskrit names, with English translations where possible. As yoga gains popularity, Sanskrit words are finding their way into common usage among yoga practitioners. Understanding these terms will help you if and when you attend classes.

Like many people, you've probably decided to take up yoga for greater fitness and flexibility, but you'll find that you get more than you bargained for. Because yoga practice is about *how* you do the postures, rather than just exercising, you may be surprised to find that, after a while, the attitudes you previously held about your mind and body have changed. As you gain more body/mind awareness and feel more peaceful, you may discover that yoga spills over into the rest of your life in unexpected ways.

The American author and philosopher Henry David Thoreau, who was also a yogi, said it brilliantly: 'Men go fishing all their lives without knowing it is not fish they are after'.

1 WHY YOGA?

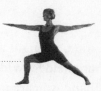

There are probably as many reasons for people being drawn to yoga as there are individuals who take it up. Yoga has successfully managed to adapt to the changing needs of yoga practitioners through the ages, including those of the nanosecond nineties.

People from all stages and all walks of life practise yoga. I know postgraduate students who use yoga to help them keep their sanity while writing PhD and master's degree theses. There are musicians who do yoga between matinee and evening orchestral perform-ances to sustain their energy levels. Some actors use yoga to foster more body awareness, give themselves a better stage presence and even help them breathe through auditions.

Some people take up yoga for the first time as children; others come to yoga late in life. A recent *Yoga Journal* article described a senior practitioner of yoga, now 100 years old, who started yoga at the age of 65 in Latvia. Another senior practitioner, an 85-year-old, was able to avoid back surgery through the improvements that daily yoga practice gave him.

No matter what your size or shape, age, gender or disposition, yoga will benefit you.

In the early days of my yoga practice, when I was a new mother, my attraction to yoga was based mainly on an emotional need for peace of mind and relaxation. (But, I must admit, I did want to shed some of my post-pregnancy weight and tone my body. It took time, but it did work!)

The great thing about yoga is that it is so adaptable and practical. If your muscles are flabby and you need to improve your tone, strength and stamina, certain yoga poses, especially if they are held for a longer period of time, will help you. If, on the other hand, you are musclebound or tense, then yoga will help you gain suppleness and joint flexibility. Body builders and triatheletes find their challenge in gaining elasticity, while those with soft bodies work to gain muscle power and endurance. Balancing your body is one of the aims of yoga.

I can't over-emphasise that the main point of yoga is not to achieve a perfect body or even a perfect pose. Although yoga does help tone and shape the body, and contributes to overall wellbeing, it offers the added value of deep relaxation and inner strength. The emphasis in yoga is not on the need to get somewhere; it's on learning to focus on the *process*, on quietening the chattering mind and tapping into the power of breathing.

Yoga is a non-competitive activity. It's non-competitive *even with yourself.* You *will* improve your health and fitness with consistent practice, but trying to force progress is counterproductive. If you are too goal-oriented, you'll tend to want to get the yoga practice over and done with, instead of learning how to work with your body and mind along the way. Being mentally and/or physically aggressive in practising yoga will ultimately limit you. One of the benefits of this type of exercise is that you learn from your strengths *and* your weaknesses. You'll miss out on the lesson of balance if you constantly push yourself beyond your body's limits. You work with your mind in yoga, so mental poise comes into this idea of balance. You will get the very utmost out of the yoga poses if you work with sensitivity and awareness.

Everyone who takes up yoga is at a different level. The good news is, if you give it your best, you will reap the same benefits as the most accomplished practitioner. This is because it is practising yoga with great awareness that's important, rather than the end result — the achievement of a perfect pose.

Benefits

The body

Yoga is a scientific method that works both systemically and systematically on every part of your body, from the skin right down to the marrow in your bones. The respiration and nervous systems, heart and blood vessels, endocrine glands, digestive organs, muscles and joints all benefit from doing yoga. It's easy to see that yoga poses affect the muscles and joints of your body, but at the same time yoga works invisibly on the internal body systems. Even as you train for flexibility, endurance, stamina and strength, exercising all of the muscle groups and joints, you are nurturing your internal organs.

When I was younger, I had quite a pushy approach to doing physical exercise, and would often feel drained rather than energised after my sessions of running or cycling. Through practising yoga, I've learned how to moderate my energy better so I can do everything I want, instead of undergoing periodic bouts of exhaustion. In my yoga practice, I balance dynamic poses with poses that recharge my batteries, and I always include a relaxation period. In the process of learning to understand my body, I've managed to heal the chronic kidney weakness that used to cause backaches and tiredness, and the irregularities I used to experience in my menstrual cycle cleared up.

You may not grow taller by doing yoga, but you'll walk and sit straighter as your overall posture improves. You may find, over time, that you will lose weight if you're too heavy, or gain weight if you're too thin, because by doing yoga regularly you will become more in touch with your body and you'll start to make healthier choices about what you eat. Some yoga poses help adjust body weight because they work on the thyroid gland, which controls metabolism.

Yoga also helps improve muscle tone. With consistent practice, it can even help develop the kind of smooth-muscled, elastic strength of a ballet dancer or gymnast.

People who do 'stress' sports, such as jogging and aerobics, frequently sustain injuries because of the need for speed of movement. Because in yoga you work your body carefully in a symmetrical and slow fashion, there is less likelihood of the strains and injuries that athletes are prone to.

One problem with many sports and exercise programs is that they build up one part of the body at the expense of another. This can eventually lead to calcification of the joints and tendon or ligament stresses. Tennis elbow is an example of this, as are knee cartilage strains and hip bursitis. Remedial yoga poses are of great help with these imbalances.

The non-athlete isn't necessarily spared injuries, either. Occupational hazards, such as the strains that office, shop and factory workers are subject to as a result of performing repetitive movements, mean that the body can become more dominant on one side than the other.

My husband, Daniel, a computer software designer, suffered wrist and shoulder pain, and numbness in his right arm. I thought this was probably a case of 'mouse-itis' (or, to be more technically accurate, carpal tunnel syndrome), and suggested he train himself to use his opposite hand on the computer mouse. Daniel included in his yoga practice some arm and shoulder stretches, and over time the problem cleared up.

Body asymmetry, whether it's structural or functional, can lead to spinal problems and wear and tear on certain joints. Musicians are very susceptible to muscle and joint strain, especially when they are not a good anatomical match for their instruments — in other words, small people playing large instruments. General stiffness and neck, shoulder and arm pains are common with musicians. When they routinely practise yoga, these problems are mitigated and hence their performances improve.

Yoga is an effective remedy when the body has been performing in a lopsided way. One of the most important techniques in practising yoga is working both sides of the body symmetrically.

People tend to identify yoga with stretching and it's true. But it's a special type of stretching called a *cross-tension stretch*. By using your muscles to anchor one part of your body, the opposing muscles stretch more effectively. It is similar to the stretching you can do at the gym with the help of machines. In yoga, however, your own body creates the resistance for a cross-tension stretch.

There are many strengthening exercises in yoga that provide balance for the postures that make you more limber. Improved muscle power is achieved by using your own body weight to create the resistance that will strengthen muscles and joints. In an advanced yoga pose such as a handstand, for example, the wrist joint is both flexed and strengthened. Any time this weight-bearing challenge is given, the joints that are effected are bathed in synovial fluid, a natural internal lubricant. When the joints are lubricated on a regular basis, they are less prone to calcification and problems such as arthritis. This effect occurs in simple poses, too, like *adho mukha svanasana* (downward-facing dog pose — page 71).

I teach remedial/therapy classes for people with injuries or medical conditions who might not otherwise be able to do yoga. The array of ailments that respond favourably to the yoga postures, breathing and relaxation is impressive. Yoga benefits people with arthritis, scoliosis and other back conditions, osteoporosis, high blood pressure, asthma, menstrual difficulties and general stress problems. Many physiotherapists, chiropractors and osteopaths recommend yoga to those who need further rehabilitation for injuries and structural imbalances. Since yoga works so well on the immune system, AIDS patients can be helped, as can people who suffer from chronic fatigue syndrome.

The mind

One of the mental benefits of practising yoga is an improvement in your ability to concentrate. This comes from focusing your mind on aligning your posture as correctly as possible and ensuring evenness in your breathing — in other words, from being more in your body than in your head. Mental distractions and obsessive thinking come to a standstill as a result of concentrating on your body and your breath. Even doing 15 or 20 minutes of only standing poses helps you focus your attention.

When you are able to hold your focus on one thing for some time, all 'mind chatter' is eliminated. This is one of the principal goals of yoga as outlined in the *Yoga-Sutras*, the definitive text on yoga (discussed in Chapter 2), which encourages 'the cessation of the fluctuations of the mind'.

We've all had the experience of our minds behaving like continuously spinning tape loops — analysing, judging, evaluating, commenting, premeditating, rehashing the past, fantasising and generally trying to figure everything out. We exhaust ourselves with the relentlessness of it all. Being able to create a deep internal focus helps to stop your mind in its tracks. When your mind is quieter, you become more aware of how your mind works and of your mental and emotional tendencies. Most of us are always thinking of the future or the past, rarely the present. Focusing on your body and your breathing brings you back to the present. This in-the-moment focus you get from doing yoga trains you to deal with stress. You are able to cope with the symptoms of stress as soon as they arise in your body, because you've developed the ability to tune in to every single adjustment you make to your body in your yoga postures.

Many people say that yoga helps their ability to concentrate on their work, and this is especially true for students. Students today are spending long hours studying for exams and working and playing at computers. These students have much tighter bodies than one would expect of people their age. While they often have to work hard at regaining their flexibility, they absolutely shine when it comes to doing yoga relaxation. They seem to be even more responsive to the relaxation than adults and thrive on the opportunity to let go.

The mental space yoga relaxation gives young people is invaluable, because it is a respite from daily stresses. It's enough for teenagers to have to contend with the emotional and physical changes of adolescence, let alone the pressure-cooker atmosphere of end-of-school exams and assessments. Yoga relaxation offers a chance for teenagers to centre themselves, because in relaxation poses there are no demands of any kind — no expectations either from themselves or from others. It is, literally, a breathing space.

The habit of stress that is developed as a teenager becomes more entrenched in adulthood. Adults who take yoga classes because they want the exercise are delighted to experience the relaxation period at the end of a yoga class. It is a transformative experience which leads many adult students to make minor shifts in favour of de-stressing the rest of their lives. (See Chapter 6 for more information on stress reduction.)

The emotions

Most people who practise yoga experience some shift in their moods, even from the beginning of a practice to the end. Part of this shift comes from the focusing of attention, part from consciously breathing while moving and stretching, and part from the special way yoga works on the internal systems of the body.

I've seen women who are experiencing premenstrual or menstrual tension begin their yoga practice feeling exhausted or irritable and finish feeling completely restored and poised.

Transitions from stressed-out to euphoric are most noticeable in my city evening classes, which I've nicknamed 'the rush-to-relax classes'. The harried business folk who arrive completely wound-up like tightly coiled springs usually leave looking younger, with an inner glow that comes from more than just exercise.

Your posture and breathing *do* affect your moods. It's almost impossible to feel happy or energetic when your body is slumped or stooped. As Charlie Brown in 'Peanuts' says of his favourite depressed stance: 'The worst thing you can do is straighten up and hold your head high, because then you start to feel better!' In your yoga practice, as you open your chest and stretch your spine, you'll find you are breathing more and, as a consequence, feeling more vital. As you improve your posture, you'll look more assured and purposeful, too.

The different yoga poses and sequences of poses have particular effects. *Surya namaskar*, the salute to the sun cycle (pages 76–77), and the standing poses are energising and strengthening. The sitting poses are pacifying and the lying poses are restful. Upside-down poses are stimulating and backbends are enlivening. This means that, in any given practice period, you can modulate how you wish to feel, to a certain extent, by which poses and which combinations you do. For instance, when you practise the poses that fall into the category of backbends, you may get a feeling of energy or even elation, because you are exercising your body in unfamiliar yet beneficial ways. Stretching the front of the body creates a huge chest opening and more lung space for the breath. The kidneys are compressed while you're holding the pose and, when you release the pose, the organs are flushed out with fresh circulation of blood. In the process, the adrenal glands are stimulated, much like getting a coffee hit without the negative effects of caffeine.

Apart from the ways yoga postures can affect how you feel, a perhaps unexpected emotional benefit comes from the commitment to do something good for yourself. When you undertake a regular activity that you know to be good for you, such as yoga practice, you are declaring to yourself that you are committed to and responsible for your own health. As your all-over wellbeing improves from doing yoga, your self-esteem and confidence begin to grow, too. You develop not only physical muscles but what is called in corporate parlance 'muscles of pro-activity'.

For me, creating a regular yoga discipline carried the most surprising, far-reaching results. It helped me develop self-assurance. Starting yoga as a 27-year-old mum, I never dreamed I would be so challenged and nourished by yoga, let alone end up teaching classes and training teachers, founding a yoga school or writing a book.

The spiritual side

I hesitate to mention the word 'spiritual' for fear of alienating any readers or causing your eyes to glaze over! I do believe, though, that in modern Western society, we have become spiritually bereft. We have lost touch with many of the things that really matter.

We may have grown up with certain religious practices and then dropped them, throwing the Bible out with the bathwater. We may feel inspired and soothed by nature and yet, for whatever reason, spend all our time in the city. Work, for so many of us, takes precedence over spending time with ourselves; being quiet and contemplative carries a very low priority.

My yoga practice is my time for solitude. I practise for about one and a half hours a day, five to six days a week (although when I was a beginner, I would just practise for 20 or 30 minutes a day). As I quietly practise the postures, I concentrate on being in my body and breath. Even if I am tremendously busy, too busy for the postures, I will give highest priority to my 10–20 minutes of relaxation, the time for my body to be completely relaxed and my mind at rest.

F. Scott Peck, who wrote *The Road Less Travelled*, as well as many other inspiring books, was asked how he managed to achieve so much each day. He said, 'Because I spend two hours every day doing nothing'.

It may appear that 'nothing' is going on in yoga relaxation poses, but this sort of centring time is such a different experience from what most of us do throughout the day and night, that it can be thoroughly transformative. I believe the ability to relax is an art and that it requires practice to become proficient at it.

Truly deep relaxation is unknown territory for many people and it brings us closer to our spiritual nature. When we surrender to deep relaxation, the experience can be like stepping through a doorway into our innermost being. This may not be what attracted you to yoga in the first place, and relaxing may be unfamiliar to you, but keep an open mind, because deep relaxation is a powerful experience.

When I first started yoga, I was practising yoga relaxation

regularly at a particularly stressful time of my life. On one occasion I had a deep experience of letting go, physically and emotionally. Lying there quietly at the end of my relaxation period, I felt tears of relief rolling down my cheeks. At the same time, I had a startling realisation: what had been holding me together was my tension! I wanted to be able to let go, but I was afraid of what was, for me, an unaccustomed feeling of surrender. Fortunately, I was able to let my body soften and relax even more, and I began to feel the first intimations of what life would be like without the pressures of continuously driving myself all the time. I discovered that I didn't need tension to get along in life.

This experience motivated me to take this relaxed way of being into my everyday activities. I began to let it flow into all the compartments of my life, such as meetings with my business partner and discussions with my accountant. I looked forward to my yoga relaxation as a time to practise letting go at deeper and deeper levels.

Over the past 17 years, I have taught countless people the yoga relaxation, many of whom say it has changed the course of their lives. This is because when you profoundly relax, you are not just letting go of tightness in muscles, ligaments and tendons, but gradually letting loose the bindings of the ego. The way we characteristically hold tension in our muscles can reflect a defensive stance. In yoga relaxation, each time you are able to let go of this holding-in of the muscles, there is a corresponding letting go of the petty personality or the need to maintain an image. When you are lying down, relaxing, there's no need to be anybody special or do anything at all. It gives you the space to let go into your spiritual self. In this sense, yoga relaxation is also a door you step through into meditation. It happens in a very natural way, as a result of the internal silence and space that you give yourself in relaxation. The aim is not escape; rather, it is to take you nearer to your essential self.

The lack of connection we have with ourselves most commonly shows itself in the way we perform our work. For many people, work could be described as an 'out-of-body' experience. Sometimes this takes the form of pushing ourselves beyond our limits to satisfy the demands of employers or employees, or when we need to get a job done quickly and so sacrifice good posture. Always rushing to get somewhere, we're often tensing muscles we don't need to be using, such as the white-knuckle grip on our car steering wheels. There's a nagging internal feeling to 'hurry up', even when there's no real need to rush. We end up neglecting our physical needs and sometimes suppressing our body's signals, because we feel pressured to 'get the job done'.

We constantly extend our physical, mental and emotional limits to meet deadlines and to be more successful. We are working longer hours for less money. What eventually happens is that we lose our capacity to push constantly ahead and we burn out.

By making a regular practice of yoga, you become more aware of your body and begin to deal with tension as it arises. You take the time to connect with yourself, balancing and healing as you practise.

Something profound happens when we reconnect with our bodies and our breathing on a regular basis. When you routinely practice yoga, it is like a continual homecoming; you *are* at home and more comfortable in your body. You're more sensitive to the things that really matter: health, energy and inner peace. Of course, fostering these qualities doesn't preclude being accomplished in the world. Fitness, vitality and equanimity are the very bedrock of long-term success, and enhance your ability to produce results.

The attitudes you develop in long-term yoga practice will permeate many aspects of your life. The fact that you are able to be present and that you feel better on so many different levels will affect your family and friends, work and recreation. You will show grace under pressure in all aspects of daily living. You will discover there's more to yoga than physical prowess. Your connections with the world will become more harmonious, and thus the practice will not only benefit you, but the planet as a whole.

2 WHAT IS YOGA?

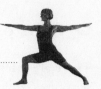

Note: If you want to begin your yoga practice right away, skip this section and jump ahead to 'Getting started' on page 29. However, if you want to understand your practice as part of the 'big picture' of yoga, read on, and you'll see that the picture is very big indeed.

The word 'yoga' comes from the Sanskrit root, *yuga*, which means 'yoke', a word that implies the joining of two things, a union. The ultimate purpose or goal of yoga is usually understood to be the joining of the individual self, or personality (*atman*), with the universal self, or the divine (*brahman*). Yoga is a path for healing the split between body, mind and spirit.

The spiritual smorgasbord that results from the many modern interpretations of this age-old discipline makes it easy to lose sight of this original healing meaning of yoga: union. Yoga 'purists' take the moral high ground of a very narrow and traditional interpretation of yoga and vie with the yoga 'revisionists', whose aim is to make their expression of yoga unrestricted and ultra-contemporary. The opposition of the two views has unfortunately created a kind of 'yoga politics'.

However, the resilience and diversity of this ancient tradition has insured that yoga has been able to adapt through changing conditions and cultures over the last 3000 years. If you want to confine yoga to a simple definition, you'll have your work cut out for you, because yoga is much too big a concept to squeeze into any old pigeonhole. Let's take a look at the big yoga picture.

Origins of yoga

There are references to yoga in the earliest of the ancient Indian scriptures, called the *Vedas*. These Vedic teachings, consisting of hymns, philosophy and rules, contributed to the great body of subsequent classical Indian literature. One of the main Vedic works is called *Upanishads*, which consists of treatises on the nature of the universal soul.

The great historical epics, *Ramayana* and *Mahabharata,* include discourses on philosophy and morality, and tell stories about the various incarnations of God.

The *Mahabharata* is an epic saga that is still performed in India and Indonesia. Peter Brooks, the famous English director, did a version for stage and film that creatively presents the *Mahabharata*'s timeless themes in a form suitable for Western audiences.

Contained in the *Mahabharata* is the *Bhagavad Gita* (Song of the Lord), which is a dialogue between God (Lord Krishna) and his devotee Arjuna, a warrior chief. Arjuna is about to go into battle and his resolve is shaky. He and Krishna discuss the different aspects of yoga, including *karma yoga, jnana yoga* and *bhakti yoga.* Although the story is ancient, the *Bhagavad Gita* is currently read and revered by millions in the east. The issues it deals with are still very topical: one's duty in life, what it takes to live ethically, the right relationship to have with regard to worldly attachments, and how to quiet the mind. All the questions are dealt with from the standpoint of the yogic big picture; in other words, what is best for one's soul.

The most influential guidelines on yoga are collected in the *Yoga-Sutras* (aphorisms), written by the Indian sage Patanjali in the 1st or 2nd century AD. The *Yoga-Sutras*, also known as the *Yoga of Eight Limbs* (*Astanga yoga*), influenced all the subsequent treatises on yoga. Patanjali's great contribution was that he gathered together the knowledge and techniques of yoga from many sources, and turned this collective knowledge into a clearly defined and systematised discipline. Up until this time, the information was conveyed by word of mouth from teachers to their disciples.

Tree of yoga

The breadth of yoga is often illustrated by the image of a tree with eight branches. The yogic path is very well mapped out, and is called *astanga*, meaning 'eight-limbed'.

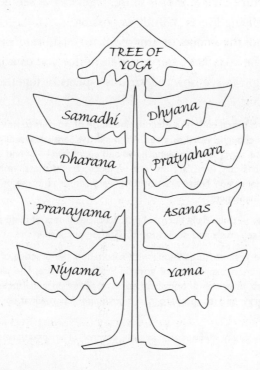

Some of the stereotypical associations with the word yoga are meditation, relaxation, contrived postures, austerity, chanting or altered states of consiousness ('bliss' states). These are all valid expressions of yoga; parts of the yoga tree. In learning yoga, you might never be interested in practising *dharana* (one-pointed concentration), but you might be very drawn to the *asanas* (the physical practice of postures). Someone who wouldn't want to come anywhere near a yoga pose may instead prefer to meditate all day long.

I couldn't conceive of sitting still long enough to meditate (let alone do relaxation) in the early days of my yoga practice, but now I've developed more patience for it. If I'd been presented with the *yama* (moral code) of yoga when I started, I would have rebelled. Now these rules make more sense, because I see how they contribute to living life as skilfully as possible.

It is beyond the scope of this book to elaborate on all the branches of the yoga tree, but it is helpful for you as a new yoga student to begin to see how the various aspects fit together.

1 *Yama* sets out a moral code, the essential intention of which is to not harm any being through thought, word or deed. Although the Sanskrit words for these rules — *ahimsa, satya, asteya, brahmacharya* and *aparigraha* — sound unfamiliar to us, they basically translate as non-violence, truthfulness, non-stealing, chastity and non-greed. These are obviously very similar to some of the great religious commandments.

2 *Niyama* relates to one's daily personal practices: cleanliness of mind and body, contentment, self-study and dedication to God or our higher self.

3 *Asanas* are the yoga postures. Along with meditation, the practice of *asanas* is the most common expression of yoga in Western culture. The aim of this discipline is to bring mind, body and spirit together in a balanced way, to generate energy and to prepare the body/mind for meditation and self-transcendence.

4 *Pranayama* is simply defined as 'breath control'. The practitioner works

on making the breath as deep and as rhythmical as possible, to foster tranquillity and calm the nervous system. The Chinese call *prana* 'chi', the Japanese 'ki', and certain Western psychotherapists call it 'bio-energy'.

To be precise, the word *prana* actually means more than just the breath or the air that we breathe. A better interpretation would be 'life force' or 'vital energy', and this includes physical senses, mental abilities and all the energy of the universe. In practising *pranayama*, one is better able to understand the energetic nature of the universe.

5 *Pratyahara* aims to discipline all the senses (touch, taste, smell, sight and hearing) in order to develop powers of concentration and meditation. This is done by withdrawing the senses so they are not aroused by external stimulation, thus creating a state of deep, internal stillness. The yoga relaxation is an approximation of this state, when the practitioner is able to successfully internalise the senses.

6 *Dharana* is the concentration achieved by training the mind to focus on a particular point or object, which leads to a deep sense of 'centredness' in the body. A *mantra* (sacred prayer) can be used as the object of focus; for example, repeating with devotion the Sanskrit sacred syllable, *aum*.

7 *Dhyana* is meditation. The ability to concentrate practised in *dharana* fosters the merging of body, breath, mind and all the aspects of the personality into one single state of being. The important element here is achieving a state of concentration in which the mind takes on aspects of the divine (compassion, serenity, detatchment, understanding) through continuous devotion.

8 *Samadhi* is absolute bliss, the ultimate goal of yoga. Meditator, meditation and the object mediated on, all lose their individual qualities and form a single vision of the universe. The practitioner in this state of supreme bliss is completely alert, but with the mind and senses at rest. It is a state of profound silence.

The various branches of the yoga tree may seem separate, but in fact they are basically interrelated. One obvious example of this is that *asana* practice (physical discipline of the body) is affected by practising *pranayama* (control of breath), and vice versa. How you practise *asanas* and *pranayama* is influenced by *yama* and *niyama*. These are the branches of yoga that are nicknamed the 'shalts' and 'shalt nots', personal practices that encourage everyday discipline and morality.

Ideally, the more you refine your practice of all the branches of yoga, the more they carry you towards a higher state of awareness, as manifested by mind, body and spirit all being in a state of harmony.

Many years ago, when I was first presented with the 'eight limbs' of yoga, I found it hard to relate to most aspects of the 'tree'. However, I now realise that it is the very breadth of the branches and the depth of the roots of the tree that invite and challenge us to keep growing in the discipline of yoga. This appeal is there long after our hamstrings have loosened up, our abdominal muscles have been strengthened and our brows have become unfurrowed.

Yoga is compelling because it is a whole and complete practice, even though it has so many aspects. Through *yamas* and *niyamas* (the moral code and individual practices), we are encouraged to have a reverential approach to the discipline. Through the *asanas* and *pranayama*, we cleanse and strengthen the body and mind, which is an expression of self-respect. The gifts of the meditative disciplines are contentment and bliss.

Experience has shown that it is possible to work on only the first five branches of the tree of yoga. These concepts reflect qualities of being that are commonly associated with yoga discipline: integrity, vitality, awareness, compassion, clarity and peacefulness. These qualities are quite practical and are an integral part of the practice of the postures, as well as a training for life. The last three branches of the tree (*dharana, dhyana* and *samadhi*) are the fruits of the practice, a kind of developmental gift when the student has attained a high level of awareness.

Yoga in the West

The big three teachers

Current popular expressions of yoga are *Iyengar yoga*, *Astanga yoga*, and *Desikachar yoga* (or *viniyoga*), all of which have a strong emphasis on *hatha yoga*, the practice of the postures.

These three styles stem originally from the tremendously influential Indian teacher, Sri T. Krishnamacharya (1888–1989), who taught B.K.S. Iyengar, K. Pattabhi Jois and T.K.V. Desikachar.

To describe Krishnamacharya's accomplishments would fill a book. Suffice to say that he and these three teachers he trained are hugely responsible for yoga's revival and spread in the West.

The yoga developed by B.K.S. Iyengar of Pune, India, is known to be demanding in the way it emphasises attention to detail, and symmetry and precision of alignment in the postures. Specialised props are used extensively in this practice. Students are expected to be very keen and absolutely dedicated to their yoga.

K. Pattabhi Jois of Mysore, India, teaches a particularly rugged method which he calls *Astanga yoga*. It is distinguished by *ujjayi* (strong breathing), accentuating a flow of postures that usually gets the practitioner sweating profusely in no time at all. One aim of this style is to generate enough heat to cleanse the body of impurities; another is to break down any rigidity in the body, and to build strength and stamina. The *Astanga* student progresses along designated levels of degrees (somewhat like the 'belts' a martial artist works to attain), from the first stage (primary level) through to the sixth stage (advanced level).

T.K.V. Desikachar of Madras, India, Krishnamacharya's son, prefers to teach students individually, with just four or five gentle postures assigned initially. The student is given a written sequence to practise, and only when these poses are mastered will more be given. *Pranayama* (breath control) and chanting are usually included as part of the sequence.

All three of these teachers have strong personalities and often those who study yoga with them model their teaching style on them.

Modern expressions of yoga

Part of the reason that yoga has been subjected to such profound adaptation, expansion and mutation in the West is, I believe, because of the accelerating complexities of modern society. Yoga has an inherent pliancy that allows it to be applied in diverse situations and to fit into new surroundings.

The mental picture of a yoga tree holds up pretty well, because a tree is alive and relatively stationary; some parts are growing and others are dying off. The actual yoga tree is, as I've said, spreading day by day and branching off in some unexpected directions.

One new development, which began in New York, is called Power Yoga, a very physical type of yoga. It's a catchy name, but one that I find difficult to reconcile with one of the aims of yoga, the transcendence of ego! Nevertheless, it's proven to be a popular speciality.

Another innovative application of yoga is being used by counsellors involved in drug and alcohol rehabilitation programs. I have met a number of people in recovery whose lives have been changed by including yoga as a major part of their daily routine. Practising yoga allows them to reduce tension, eliminate toxins and heal the nervous system. One rehabilitation centre in the United States uses meditation, breathing exercises and special yoga routines to facilitate healing and give a natural high. It claims an impressive 91 per cent success rate.

A Japanese amalgam of yoga, created by Masahiro Oki, is called

Oki Yoga. I've nicknamed it 'kamikaze' yoga because it is a very intense form — blending martial arts, Western exercise and therapeutic movements — that pushes you to your physical limits.

Some of the yoga tree's branches have withered and dropped by the wayside of our modern culture, such as the practice of asceticism (including *brahmacharya* or sexual continence). Another branch, *tantra*, seems to have supplanted asceticism.

Yoga has infiltrated the corporate world with the offering of regular yoga classes for staff. Stress-management courses train office workers in what are basically relaxation and meditation techniques.

The Internet has plenty of yoga home pages. Recently, I stumbled across a research paper called 'The Yoga of Management'. In another search I found some yoga sequences on menstruation.

Many doctors are adapting yoga practices for their patients. I know one Western GP who teaches his heart-risk patients biofeedback techniques to lower their heart rates. He also sells them 'neti pots', which are devices for helping patients relieve sinusitis with nasal saltwater treatments.

This huge variety of yoga practices may be thought by yoga purists to be degrading to this ancient discipline. I prefer to think of all the innovation that is occurring as something that helps to bring balance wherever it's needed. Even in India, yoga's original home, life is not as simple as it used to be, and many yogic traditions are being left behind and/or modernised.

It is important when looking for a teacher to find one you are comfortable with. Sometimes students are put off yoga because the style or the teacher didn't suit them. Choose a style of yoga that suits what you want to achieve, and a teacher who teaches with love and caring.

The yoga approach is experiential, meaning you are encouraged to verify your own experience, not simply subscribe to dogma. Therefore, it's important to exercise your choice. You may even find that what works best for you is an integral yoga approach — blending various alternatives that serve your needs. When you commit to following a certain path, have a questioning mind and test the practice through your own experience.

These are the various possible paths:

HATHA YOGA *Hatha yoga* (the approach used in this book) is a popular path because of the tremendous interest we now have in health and fitness. It comprises practices for controlling the body and mind. One goal is to increase *prana* (the flow of energy) through the spinal column by practising the *asanas* (postures). Seated postures, in particular, facilitate the stability and serenity that is required for meditation.

I'd like to say more about the *hatha yoga* path, because it's more widely pursued in the West than the other disciplines.

A big attraction to *hatha yoga* is its physicality. People want to look and feel good. But people also want to be doing an *intelligent* form of physical exercise.

Yoga is not just an exercise routine or physical therapy, but ultimately something more like meditation-in-action. Yoga practice can become, in time, a subtle dance of awareness between the action of the *asanas* and the stillness of a peaceful mind. This happens when the student is able to maintain a continuous dialogue between body and mind. It is no small feat. The ability to be aware and absorbed in the poses involves other disciplines — *pratyahara*, *dharana* and *dhyana* (explained in the 'Tree of Yoga' on page 17), those aspects of yoga that are usually associated with meditation.

My own starting point in doing yoga was the physical side — toning and stretching muscles, ligaments and tendons. After a while, it dawned on me that I also needed to stretch and integrate my intellect as I was doing each pose, and, in time, my practice became more of a meditation-in-action. As I was learning to keep my mind totally focused on the poses, I experienced each of them more fully.

A mature yoga practice outwardly looks quite physical, but inwardly there is an unfolding of awareness. You grow spiritually, as a result.

RAJA (ROYAL) YOGA is the path for those who feel called to practise what is generally considered the classical path of yoga — inner and outer self-control. *Raja* practitioners are in the world but not of it, and have strength of character and a calm, meditative mind, which they achieve by eliminating the restlessness of the mind.

KARMA YOGA *Karma* yogis practice the discipline of 'right action' — the work they do *is* their practice. They perform their work selflessly and mindfully, dedicating it as service to others. This path suits a dynamic person, but one who is not attached to working for a reward. Rather than thinking of quick profit, the karma yogi thinks of the long term, and is not attached to the fruits of his or her labour. It doesn't matter what expression work takes, paid or unpaid, in the home or outside of it, the work is done as a spiritual offering.

TANTRA YOGA is becoming increasingly popular in the West, because of the common interpretation that tantra relates mainly to the practice of certain sexual rituals. However, this is not an altogether correct assumption. *Tantra* is actually meant to be a path of self-transcendence whereby ceremonies and rituals are used to celebrate the Divine in ourselves and others. It is a discipline that suits a person who enjoys ceremony and uses it to express the philosophy that the Divine is a part of our ordinary life.

BHAKTI YOGA is the path of self-transcending devotion or all-embracing love of the Divine, which is seen to be part of every person and every thing. *Bhakti yoga* is for those whose temperaments are worshipful and who seek to cultivate an open heart. Some people think *bhakti* is an easy approach, but for it to bear spiritual fruit, the practice must emanate from pure and heartfelt practice.

JNANA YOGA is the path of discernment. The yogi or yogini (male or female practitioner) learns to distinguish between what is real and what is unreal — the difference between true happiness and fleeting pleasure. This is the path of the sage who understands that spiritual progress depends on dispelling the illusion that we are only our bodies and our minds. This path calls to those with a rational mind and a high degree of intuition and discernment.

Sanskrit — the language of yoga

Sanskrit derives from the Indo-Aryan languages, roots that linguists are inclined to believe English and Sanskrit have in common. The oldest Indo-Aryan writing dates from the 14th century BC. During the 4th century BC, Indian grammarians worked to refine one of the archaic dialects, which then became known as Sanskrit (meaning 'polished' or 'perfected'). Sanskrit developed into the official language of religion, as well as being used in a vast array of philosophical, narrative, lyric, dramatic and technical writing. Patanjali's *Yoga-Sutras*, dated between 400 and 200 BC, was written in Sanskrit.

Sanskrit terminology is used more frequently now to describe the yoga poses than it was when I first started yoga. My yoga teacher thought it was elitist to use the Sanskrit words. But we live in cosmopolitan times and using Sanskrit means we'll be understood by yoga students worldwide.

You may have some difficulty at first getting a grasp of the terminology, but Sanskrit terms do add a level of skill to yoga practice, as each of the names is so specific and reflects the symbolism of each pose. Each name has a symbolic meaning, which may represent geometric shapes, creatures or features from nature, or heroes and sages of history or myth. Therefore, the names themselves carry great power because they engage our imagination. Each time we perform an *asana*, we are seen to be creating a symbolic gesture with our body and our mind. This experience creates a link between the yoga practitioner and the energy behind the symbol. We can identify with the stability of a tree (*vrksha*), the suppleness of the monkey-god, *Hanuman*, or with the warrior energy of *Virabhadra*.

By learning the names of the poses, you learn more about the Hindu gods and Indian history and mythology. This helps you to understand the rich culture from which yoga springs.

3 GETTING STARTED

Motivation

The motivation for practising yoga is a very individual thing. It comes from what *you* wish to get out of it.

I had fun doing yoga from the very first time I tried it, and this kept me interested and looking forward to the time I set aside for practice. If you know the fun and pleasure of being in your body in an aware way, you don't meet as much resistance in the practice — even with the challenging poses. As you do more yoga and it becomes an integral part of your life, you will find that you welcome your practice periods.

Many people are motivated by the fact that they feel better after each practice session. This is enough to keep them practising yoga on a regular basis — especially when their friends tell them they look better, or their children say they like them more because they're more relaxed. It is very encouraging to know that if you start your practice feeling tense and perhaps with your shoulders right up around your ears, you're likely to finish feeling balanced, energetic and more in touch with yourself.

It is extremely motivating to feel your body becoming stronger and more supple week by week, which goes against the tide of what we perceive as the effects of 'normal' ageing. I was quite amazed to find that, generally speaking, the high school students to whom I taught yoga were way behind my level of fitness, strength and flexibility, although I'm three times their age. Unfortunately, what we still accept as the 'norm' as we get older is based on what kind of shape our parents, grandparents and other elders are in, and not looking at what's possible in terms of doing a lifetime exercise regime.

A popular incentive for doing yoga is to de-stress and find a more balanced lifestyle. There's a pitfall with this approach, however. If your reason for taking up yoga is to develop a more relaxed lifestyle, and you notice that the time you set aside is constantly eroded by personal and/or business emergencies, to reach your goal will take conscious management. You may have to start being more selfish about your time. I find it helpful to make an appointment with myself in my diary, giving top priority to my yoga practice time.

Another factor which motivates many people to practise yoga regularly is that, for the first time in their lives, they are able to manage the chronic aches and pains they've been putting up with, just by doing some basic yoga stretches. It is especially motivating when people discover that if they miss out on a few sessions, the symptoms start coming back. This makes the choice between whether to continue spending time and money on the chiropractors, osteopaths, and physiotherapists, or whether simply to do your own yoga practice, remarkably clear-cut. These days, patients are often instructed by their GP or alternative medical practitioner to take up yoga. The aim is to reinforce and sustain the balancing of the body that's been achieved, and to wean patients off the need for constant treatment.

The main thing that keeps me coming back to my yoga practice is the self-nurturing that it provides. I am a very busy person and come in contact with a great number of people every day. My practice session 'feeds' me, and I seldom feel depleted or overwhelmed by my daily activities. If I do start to feel out of balance, I practice restorative poses (pages 104–108), those invaluable supported postures that soothe the nervous system and restore energy.

By setting aside a regular time for doing the postures and the yoga relaxation, I give myself a chance to touch base. This is time when I don't think about what I've read in the newspaper, or concern myself with my finances, or consider what I should cook for dinner. As a consequence of having looked after my whole being in my practice, I have new-found energy for resuming my duties, a fresher perspective and sometimes new slants on the 'old slog'.

Eventually, yoga practice becomes something you can rely on, a precious and essential part of your life because of the psychic breathing space it affords. You have a daily ritual, where you spend time by yourself, for yourself. Yoga practice is practical. The more you consistently dedicate yourself to it, the more you begin to dance to your own rhythm. As Michael Leunig, the cartoonist, says in the introduction to *A Common Prayer* about practising a daily ritual: 'Each time it occurs something important is revitalised and strengthened. The garden is watered'.

Potential obstacles

In this section, we'll take a realistic look at some of the obstacles to practising that I've encountered — what might be in your way when you notice that the garden isn't being watered.

Let's face it: organising and establishing a yoga practice at home isn't necessarily easy. The reason why some people only ever come to yoga classes and don't practice on their own is that, in classes, they're led by the teacher, while at home, they actually have to think about how and what they're doing.

Learning in a class *is* very helpful. However, I've discovered that the people who get the most out of yoga don't only go along to classes. Those who progress are the ones who put more of themselves into their yoga, through a regular practice at home. Progress occurs with a relatively small, but regular, investment of your time and energy. As you would expect, the more you put into practising, the more you get out of yoga.

It pays to have a personal yoga practice, too, for those times when you just can't get to classes, because you're on holidays, or travelling for business reasons, or in an area where there are no yoga teachers available. When you have firmly established your own yoga practice, you'll never miss out on having energy, clarity and peace, wherever you are.

Classes help by providing valuable knowledge, but personal practice gives you a deepening experience of yourself on many levels, including your capacity for self-discipline.

When you first start practising yoga, it can be difficult — you need to think about the details of the pose and work out the logistics of it, and think about your breath. This applies to learning any new activity. Eventually, you will stay focused and will become both more efficient and more intuitive in your practice.

Some of the common stumbling blocks to keeping up a regular practice are discussed below.

Lack of enthusiasm

No matter how motivated you may be initially, enthusiasm has a way of ebbing and flowing. If you find your interest in yoga has waned, you may need to think back to why you wanted to do yoga in the first place, and recreate the vision of what you want.

Renewing your interest in yoga practice will fan your enthusiasm. This done by keeping your attention on what's happening from moment-to-moment in your poses and with your breath.

When you hit a wall of boredom or lack of enthusiasm, it's a wake-up call that perhaps you have been inattentive in your practice. Since increasing your capacity for attention is one of the aims of yoga, it's an opportunity to renew your commitment to being attentive.

Doubts

You may have doubts that you're achieving the results you expected and sometimes it just takes repetition of the poses until you feel coordinated in the movements. You may feel that what worked yesterday isn't working today, or that you're 'losing it' because you can't remember what you've already learned.

Don't worry! All it takes is repetition of the poses. Patient, steady practice *will* ensure your steady progress. The best approach to yoga is to work to your limits without pushing yourself too far. If you obsess about reaching a certain standard, you miss the point of doing yoga. It's not about being perfect; yoga is a training in awareness. Notice when you're 'leaking' your energy by indulging in self-doubt and worry. Even if this has caused you to miss your practice today, don't beat yourself up about it; just make sure you practise tomorrow.

Pain

When you start doing any new exercise regime, it's not unusual to experience discomfort, soreness and even pain, and yoga is no different. But don't let that put you off. It's important to be able to understand the distinction between 'good pain' and 'bad pain'.

If you haven't exercised since you were at school and that was a *very* long time ago, it stands to reason that stretching and toning your muscles will be challenging for you. The intense sensations you may experience are likely to be 'good pain'. When you practise yoga on a regular basis, you'll also be releasing muscle tightness. Your body will open up, little by little, and the poses won't hurt so much. If you aren't particularly athletic, you are a perfect candidate for this type of exercise, because you can go at your own pace initially and build up your suppleness and strength slowly over time.

If and when you do feel sharp pain, and particularly if you can't relax and breathe through it or it lasts, this may indicate 'bad pain'. You need to stop and check that you're not overriding your body's limits. Generally, pain can be alleviated by backing off, and when you do, you get some valuable feedback about whether you were being mentally aggressive. For example, if your neck feels uncomfortable after a session, notice if you tend to contract your neck and hunch your shoulders as you practice.

Your anatomy and the pose need to match up; if you superimpose your image of the perfect pose on your body and your body is not ready for it yet, warning bells of pain will announce loud and clear that you're probably being too goal-oriented. You are being given very useful feedback about trying to dominate your body with willpower.

The people who stay with yoga long-term are the ones who learn early on to honour their body signals. Remember that you are on a journey. You are exploring this pose in this moment, not a 'one day, some day' idealised image of a pose. You will enjoy yoga more, and will have more of yourself and your breath available, if you're not totally fixated on the destination. Working in a more tuned-in way, it's very unlikely that you'll end up damaging yourself.

Tiredness or emotional upset

It seems contrary to logic to want to exercise when feeling exhausted. However, specific restorative yoga exercises have a recharging and renewing effect. *Supta baddha konasana* (lying-down, bound-angle pose — page 105), *viparita karani* (legs-up-the-wall pose — page 106), seated forward stretches and the yoga relaxation all — especially if held for longer timings — work wonders in eliminating mental and physical fatigue.

When you do the restorative yoga sequences, the inherent restfulness of the poses allows your own natural healing ability to come to the fore. These reviving poses help overcome fatigue and jet lag, and accelerate your recovery from an illness.

From time to time, you may experience an emotional upset that comes up during your practice time. This can take the form of irritability, fear, sadness, frustration or anger. Sometimes you'll understand why you are experiencing these feelings, at other times it will be a complete mystery. Learn to observe objectively any feelings that arise in the same way you observe any physical sensations of discomfort you experience in the postures.

When I started yoga, I experienced great waves of frustration and sadness, whenever I performed a sequence of the seated forward bends. Sometimes I would finish a session crying. No one had explained to me that emotional discomfort could arise while doing yoga. Part of my upset related to discomfort I experienced as I challenged my *very* tight hamstrings. However, I recognised that there were other situations in my life where I would characteristically collapse in despair when presented with a tough challenge. Dealing with this familiar pattern when it came up in my practice eventually helped me deal with it in my life outside yoga time.

I had the opportunity to ask the yoga guru, T.K.V. Desikachar, why these upsets can happen in practice. He said it is a Western problem that relates to 'the pending file'. He meant that people in the West generally don't experience their feelings as they arise, so they are shoved into a mental 'pending file' to be dealt with later. 'Later' can sometimes be when you are quietly practising and there's the time and sensitivity for experiencing your emotions more deeply.

At times such as this, you have the opportunity to strengthen 'the observer', the part of yourself that watches you practice. Acknowledge your emotions. Be aware if any of your feelings are familiar responses to problems that arise at other times. Detached observation of your feelings will often calm them. If feelings of futility arise about poses that are difficult, put the emphasis on what you *are* able to do and don't give up.

My teacher used to correct me when I bemoaned the fact that I couldn't do forward bends by saying to me, 'You can't do them *yet!*'. Eventually I moved from a belief that I would never be able to do the poses to 'I'll give it a go' and, finally, to 'Yes, I can'.

Lack of discipline

If you believe that laziness is your problem, I'd be willing to bet my yoga mat that this is a problem that has been dogging you in other situations and for quite a long time. It may help you to think in terms of cultivating yoga practice as a new good habit, or what I call a 'positive addiction'.

A big downfall in initiating and maintaining any new activity is that we often don't do it for long enough for it to become a deeply ingrained habit. When I hear people say they're not disciplined enough to do yoga on their own, that they're too lazy, I'm tempted to challenge their use of the word 'discipline'. My computer thesaurus tells me discipline is synonymous with control, rules and punishment! For me, discipline equals learning. To learn anything takes repetition and the willingness to persevere.

Try not to become obsessed with whether or not you have the

requisite discipline. Rather, put all that wasted mental energy into setting aside a period of time to practise your yoga, and stick to it. This amounts to making an agreement with yourself to do yoga regularly — a month's duration is perhaps a good initial objective. Then, you just go ahead and do what you said you were going to do.

If it sounds too easy, it is! It's your mind that makes it complicated by generating reasons *not* to do what you set out to do. Reasonably speaking, you *don't* have time, you *are* too busy, you *are* feeling tired and you *do* have a headache. This is the job of the mind, to be 'reasonable', but our minds are not always our best friends, and it works well to turn off the mind chatter and 'just do it'. You'll find that the reasons for not having done your practice usually disappear by the time you finish your practice, and instead of the low-grade anxiety you might have experienced from procrastinating, you experience a feeling of accomplishment. This adds up, in small increments, until you feel more confident in your ability to practise yoga. And besides, during your practice, you're consistently receiving all the good feelings, such as fitness, vitality and tranquillity.

If you can learn to harness your mind in this way for doing your yoga practice, you can apply the same skill to practising your singing, your golf swing, your ballroom dance steps, your touch-typing — absolutely anything!

Too little time

Since 'too little time' is one of the most common excuses I hear for not practising, I'll repeat the old maxim: *everyone has the same 24 hours in a day.* If you can't imagine where to find the time to give to yoga practice, it may be that you're unaware of where your time goes. I suggest that, over a few days, you look at how you *do* spend your time, and write down what you do at 30-minute intervals from the time you wake up until the time you go to sleep. It is more than likely that you'll discover a bracket of 15–30 minutes that you could commit to yoga.

Through practising yoga, you will end up with more energy and may find you require less sleep. Rather than sacrificing your valuable time, you will have instead acquired a positive new habit, and maybe even created more free time in your busy life.

What you need

Clothing and space

For maximum comfort while you are practising, wear clothing that has enough 'give' without being too baggy, to enable you to move and stretch easily. You can wear a T-shirt and shorts in warmer weather, or a tracksuit when the weather is cooler. Leotards and tights are a popular choice with many women. It is best to be barefoot so that you won't slip and so that your feet are more sensitive to the ground you are standing on.

As you will be breathing more than you usually do, make sure you are in a well-ventilated space. One well-known Indian teacher advises that students practise in a clean, airy place, with no noise or insects, a set-up that's easier for us to ensure in the West than I found it to be in India!

Turn down the bell on your phone and turn off your mobile phone and fax machine. This is *your* time, so don't let all those electronic intrusions rob you of your focus and peace of mind.

Equipment

It is possible to practise yoga with no equipment at all. Some people like this pristine approach because it is straightforward and the practice just flows. It's entirely up to you. However, I find that having some basic equipment is helpful, not only because it makes the practice easier, but because you tend to take what you're doing more seriously if you have the proper tools.

You can find most of the equipment you need (or some creative alternatives) around the house, except perhaps for a yoga mat. Purchasing a yoga mat is money well spent, especially if you buy one of the thin types made from non-skid material, commonly called 'sticky mats'. Since you can't slip on these mats, your feet can grip and work more strongly, especially in the standing poses. The mat provides a softer place when you're lying down, too, especially if your physique is of the bonier type. A mat also helps delineate your yoga space, much like your desk helps compartmentalise your work.

You can use props, if you wish, to make certain poses more attainable, which is encouraging for beginners. Props are especially good for you if your body tends to be very tight or if you have any injuries. You are not always going to be completely comfortable in a pose, but you'll find it is very distracting if you have to tense up so much that your body is more contracted when you finish a pose than when you started! When there is a prop for support, you are able to relax to a certain extent because the mind gets the message that you aren't doing it all on your own.

These are the props that, in my experience, are the most useful. They are available through some yoga schools.

1 A soft strap, about 2 m long and 5 cm wide, to help you catch hold of your foot in lying-down leg stretches and forward bends.

2 A wooden block, about 8 cm x 13 cm x 23 cm, or a stack of similarly proportioned books (tied together), for resting your hand on in standing poses.

3 One or two firm twin-size blankets for sitting postures and for the relaxation.

4 A folding chair or any straight-backed chair, with a flat seat.

5 An eye bag (a small rectangular cloth bag filled with sand or grain), or a soft cloth or scarf, to cover the eyes for the restorative poses and the relaxation.

Guidelines

1 Exercise caution in taking up yoga practice if you have any health problems. The postures are not really substitutes for professional advice or care, so if you think or know you have a condition that needs treatment, see a medical practitioner before starting yoga.

2 Avoid practising in direct sunlight or doing yoga directly after being in the hot sun, as you risk becoming overheated and/or dizzy.

3 If you experience pain while in a pose, consider it a warning bell. Don't just keep going if you get a sharp pain, especially if it is in the lower back, neck, hips or knees. It may be that you need to use a prop, or it may indicate that you are pushing your body too deeply, too fast and you need to back off. You are using your intelligence to go with your body, not against it.

If pain persists in a particular pose, you may need to check that your alignment is correct and make sure that you are stretching both sides of the body evenly, or check what you are doing with an experienced yoga teacher.

This question of how hard to work in the poses bears looking at in more depth. If you work too gently, you don't necessarily go deeply enough to engage your mind and body. If you work too hard, you can become exhausted and perhaps injure yourself. However you resolve this question, you will be learning a great deal about your body and your attitude.

The philosophy of 'no pain, no gain' arose in the 1980s, when aerobics classes were at their height of popularity and people who were unfit sometimes sustained injuries because they pushed their bodies too far, too fast. This philosophy is inappropriate to yoga, although that doesnt mean your yoga practice should be totally self-indulgent and 'wimpy'.

It bears repeating: yoga is all about a balanced approach to exercise, doing the very best you can, but without pushing your body past its limit. If you've been much more committed to being a couch potato in recent times than being a triathelete, you may need to go through an initial phase of discomfort as you stretch tight muscles and open rusty joints. In this phase, your body will be much more willing to cooperate and you will actually make better progress using intelligence and finesse rather than force.

4   During menstruation, women are well served by doing some particular yoga poses that make up a menstrual sequence. *Supta baddha konasana* (lying-down bound-angle pose — page 105) and the forward stretches, with your head resting on the seat of a chair or on folded blankets, are especially good for alleviating cramps and restoring vitality. How much a woman does, of course, depends entirely on her energy level at the time. If she is feeling totally drained and lacking in energy, she's better off doing nothing in the first and second day of her period, except, perhaps, the yoga relaxation. As any Zen monk would advise: it is very wise and good for us to rest when we are tired.

In some traditional societies, it is considered taboo for a woman to participate in her normal activities during her menstrual period. In our Western society, however, women would be extremely hard-pressed to take this amount of time off once a month, even if they knew it would be a lifesaver. I've found it makes a tremendous difference to do 30 minutes to an hour of restorative poses when menstruating. These postures balance and energise the body, and clarify the mind. They also help greatly with the symptoms of premenstrual tension.

5   Pregnant women are encouraged to do yoga, commensurate with their level of fitness. For women embarking on the yoga path for the first time at the outset of their pregnancy, I recommend beginning very slowly and introducing new postures gradually.

The beautiful thing about the pregnancy yoga practice is that it gives the mother-to-be regular time alone with the baby growing inside her. By setting aside this special time for yoga, she tends to be more aware of the miraculous changes occurring in her body. Each day her body looks, moves, and feels different and, in doing her yoga, she's tuned into this process with great awareness, right up to her delivery day. Poses which involve any abdominal exercises and strong twists should be avoided.

Yoga can be resumed about six weeks after giving birth.

6   It's advisable to do yoga on an empty stomach, which means you should not have eaten for about two hours before practice.

There are few things worse than the slightly bilious feeling you get, especially in any bending-forward or upside-down positions, if you exercise with a full stomach! However, if you do exercise following a meal, *virasana* (page 62) is a wonderful antidote to indigestion or flatulence, and may save you a visit to the chemist.

If you have low blood sugar, however, you may need to have a small snack about an hour before you start practising.

7 The length of time you maintain a particular yoga pose depends on your strength and stamina. After a practice session, notice if you feel tired. It may be that you are holding poses for too long or are trying too hard. Ideally, you will feel rejuvenated after practice.

The restorative poses are usually held for longer periods.

8 Keep your eyes open in the poses so you can see where to adjust your body. This helps you stay focused. However, when you're doing the restorative postures or relaxation, you may want to have your eyes closed and covered with an eye bag or soft cloth.

9 Remember to breathe going into a pose, while you're in the pose, and as you come out. Always breathe through the nostrils, not through the mouth, if possible.

If your breathing is at all strained, it usually means you are trying too hard! Another indication that you're overexerting yourself is that your eyes, jaw, throat and shoulders are tense. Just soften a little; work smarter, not harder.

10 Time yourself when you do poses that require you to work on one side of the body and then the other, to ensure you give equal time to stretching both sides of the body evenly.

11 Approach your practice with equal measures of awareness and gentleness. Treat your body with the utmost respect. It is not respectful to be aggressive with your body in your practice, but it is equally disrespectful to be lazy.

When you commit yourself to yoga, you are taking on a lifelong challenge of finding the middle ground between too little and too much. This is a new experience for many people. You learn to observe what you are doing and what your attitude is. The ability to observe with detachment is a powerful skill, because it connects you with yourself at a very deep level.

4 YOGA PRACTICE

Before beginning your yoga practice, there are a few things you need to consider: when to practise, how much you want to do, what sort of practice relates to the various seasons, cycles and your energy, how you put the poses together, and how to breathe.

To consider all these aspects encourages intelligent practice and means you'll get more satisfaction and benefits from it.

When to practise

The optimum time for you to practise will be dictated by your daily schedule. As I mentioned earlier, when I started doing yoga, I found my best (and only available) practice time was when I put my son down for his afternoon nap. So it's up to you, too, to determine the best time, although the time isn't as important as the *regularity* of practising. This is because it will help you to set a habit. In my experience, early mornings work well for most people, as you can usually find a bit of extra time in the first part of the day. Set the alarm clock a little earlier, get up and do the yoga practice before the day and your mind get too busy. Minds (I don't know why this is so, but it does seem to be universally true) are better at creating reasons why *not* to do something good for you than to *do* something good for you. Early in the morning is the ideal time to bypass this unfortunate characteristic of our minds.

By practising early in the morning you'll head off to work feeling more awake and vibrant. You will have managed, too, to set the day's dial to stress-free, even if afterwards you have to sit in rush-hour traffic, as many of us do.

After work or early in the evening is also an excellent time to practise, particularly if you have a meeting or social engagement to attend afterwards. Practising the postures and doing the relaxation will give you just the lift you need to be able to look forward to these activities, instead of being concerned about dragging yourself along or falling asleep.

Another advantage of practising yoga in the evening, especially if you are stiff, is that your body has had a chance to loosen up during the day. It is a trade-off, however, because even though your muscles will be more supple, you may feel less energetic.

It is best not to do the more dynamic poses late at night, because you'll find they charge up your energy and make it harder to fall asleep. On the other hand, if you have insomnia, some of the more soothing yoga poses, and definitely the relaxation, will help you sleep like a baby.

How much to practise

As a newcomer to yoga, you can probably manage three or four sessions a week. Obviously, a longer practice time will give you more benefits, but even doing a shorter session regularly will help build a solid habit and boost your confidence. Doing a session of 15 or 20 minutes is obviously better than nothing, and you will be surprised that you can accomplish so much in that amount of time.

It is always obvious to me when students who come to their once-a-week class at the yoga school begin to do home practice. Their level of skill and self-assurance improves enormously which, in turn, inspires them to want to practise more. There are so many benefits to be had from classroom instruction. Students are given lots of details, hands-on adjustments and correction. But home practice is what makes yoga your very own.

After you've been doing yoga for some time, you become hooked on the good effects, and you naturally want to extend the length of your practice time. When I was training to be a yoga teacher, I would often do a two-hour morning session and another two-hour session in the evening. I was so keen that sometimes I would do even more, and I definitely learned quickly this way.

Most people, even if they want to do yoga more intensively, couldn't afford this amount of time. Even now, with my family, home and business to look after, I'm careful how I organise my yoga time. Generally, I do a late afternoon practice (before I teach an evening class) and set aside about one and a half to two hours for yoga, five or six days a week.

There's no rush. Yoga is a lifelong practice. The people who go the distance, in my experience, are the ones who are realistic about how much and how often to practise. And with yoga, a little regular practice will do a surprising amount of good.

Seasons and cycles

I spoke earlier about how to adjust your practice according to a daily cycle, diurnal versus nocturnal, to be precise. It's helpful to look at a few other cycles that influence the 'what' and 'how' of your practice. The cycles a woman experiences (menstruation, pregnancy and menopause) are the most obvious ones, but all cycles, if paid attention to, help us to be more tuned in to the present moment, and in harmony with the seasons of life.

Seasons

In India, yoga is traditionally adapted to suit the extreme seasonal changes. An Indian yogi or yogini would do certain poses in the dry season and different ones in the wet season.

Nowadays, we are mostly oblivious to the rhythms of nature. When we consider modifying our practice to fit in with seasonal changes, we are re-establishing a very important link between ourselves and nature.

It's natural for us to want to do different routines in the humidity and heat of summer compared with those we do in the chilling weather of winter. When the weather feels oppressively hot, for example, I still want to be able to practise, so I do lying-down, chest-opening and restorative poses. These postures keep the body open, relaxed and cool. On the other hand, cold weather calls for us to do stronger yoga and more dynamic, warming poses and sequences, such as *surya namaskar* (salutes to the sun — page 76), which help reduce the joint and muscle stiffness we experience in winter.

In the same spirit of establishing a cyclic connection with nature, I sometimes plan my practices to fit in with the lunar cycle. I do quieter poses in the dark moon phase, building up to more intense practice in the full moon.

Age

Children can and do practice yoga. They tend to want to do everything and anything they see. If they happen to see their parents doing yoga, it's definitely 'monkey see, monkey do' time, often with very cute results.

A child's attention span is generally short, so they find it difficult to hold a pose. But with their more playful approach to yoga, children seem to explore their physical limits in a natural way. I sometimes think it was actually children who invented yoga, because it comes so easily to them. (Have you ever noticed the way infants and toddlers spontaneously do movements that look suspiciously like yoga?)

Many of the Sanskrit names for the poses translate to animal names: there are dog (*adho* and *urdhva mukha svanasana*), fish (*matsyasana*), turtle (*kurmasana*), lion (*simhasana*) and peacock (*pincha mayurasana*) poses. Identifying with a creature captures a child's ultra-active imagination right from the beginning.

As I mentioned in Chapter 1, teenagers can benefit hugely from the stability of a yoga practice, in the face of all the other changes taking place in their bodies and emotions. Adolescence and the yoga relaxation make for a perfect combination.

I've met quite a few adults who had the good fortune to learn yoga in their youth and then kept it up. They are the envy of all who take up the practice much later in life.

When people reach middle age, yoga can be an effective antidote for the midlife crisis. Let's face it, there's often plenty of scope for improving both body and mind in these middle years. For those who apply themselves to the practice of yoga in middle age, the physical and mental changes can be astounding; this is not only because of the way they regain their youthful vigour and physique, but, more importantly, because yoga helps them relate with more acceptance to the body they have right now.

Those who are in the 60-plus age category, I find particularly inspiring as yoga practitioners. Yoga is one activity that is increasingly popular among people in this age group because it retards the loss of flexibility and strength that we expect our bodies to experience as part of the ageing process. In fact, some over-60s are delighted to discover that they are able to use their bodies in ways they haven't *ever* been able to before, or perhaps haven't done since they were children. They actually manage to turn back the clock in terms of becoming more agile or energetic by practising yoga regularly.

I suppose the ultimate argument, when you come right down to it, is wouldn't you rather be ageing in a healthy, supple, fit body?

It's good practice to approach learning yoga more slowly when one is older. As you would expect with the burgeoning older population, there are now yoga videos and books that specifically address the senior market.

Older students seem to understand that it's unlikely they will master the most advanced yoga poses in their lifetimes. This makes them less competitive and more patient in their practice. They are also more open to the main purpose of doing yoga, which is to cultivate awareness and bring together body, mind and spirit. For them, the qualities of presence and wisdom that are cultivated in the practice of yoga are the crowning glory, and the improvements that they make in their levels of fitness and wellbeing are more like icing on the cake.

Menstruation

Women need to take into account when, how and what to practise, depending on exactly where they are in their menstrual cycle. A well-planned yoga sequence of special menstrual poses will usually help with the release of menses, eliminate tiredness and balance hormones.

The following poses are a boon to menstruating women and are successful in reducing premenstrual tension: *baddha konasana* (pages 64 and 105), in both the lying-back position and as a forward stretch, to help open the abdomen and pelvis, and to ease cramps and bloating; *upavistha konasana* (page 98), as a forward stretch or twist, with the buttocks against the wall and the legs resting on the wall, to help with leg aches and headaches; forward *virasana* (page 95), with the torso supported on a bolster or blankets, to help relieve lower back and sacrum ache; *paschimottanasana* (page 97) and *janu sirsasana* (page 96), with the head supported on blankets or a chair, to stretch the legs and lower back. The yoga relaxation is invaluable for reducing irritability and tension.

It's generally not recommended to do the more strenuous poses and upside-down poses where the flow of menstrual blood can be disturbed.

Pre- and post-pregnancy

Pregnancy is a great time to be doing yoga. Many women take it up for the first time during pregnancy, because it is so highly recommended in birth education courses and books. It's an intelligent and gentle way to exercise that can be done right up until the onset of labour. Pregnancy is such an individual journey that the woman must at all times look to her own comfort while practising; if poses don't feel right, it's best to leave them out. Postures that feel just fine in the first trimester of pregnancy may feel totally wrong in the last trimester.

The standing poses help a woman cultivate the stamina and strength, especially in her legs, that she will need for labour. The sitting poses, such as *baddha konasana*, (lying back and forward stretch), and *upavistha konasana* (splits) facilitate flexibility and openness, particularly in the hips and the pelvic floor. The emphasis on aware breathing in yoga is a vital tool for all the labour stages. If the mother-to-be has learned the lesson of letting go and breathing through difficult yoga poses, she'll be better prepared to face each painful contraction. If she's learned to relax in *savasana* (page 108), she'll make good use of the respites between uterine contractions to rest and conserve her energy.

Here's a simple sequence for pregnant women:

- *baddha konasana* (page 64), for 5 minutes (or longer);
- *virasana* (page 62), for 2–3 minutes;
- standing poses, such as *trikonasana* (page 80), *virabhadrasana II* (page 82), and *parsvakonasana* (page 84), with the back against a wall for support, two repetitions, holding the position for 10–15 breaths;
- *janu sirsasana* (page 96), two repetitions, holding the pose for 2 minutes each side;
- *paschimottanasana* (page 97), for 3–5 minutes (keeping the chest well lifted to make space for the baby);
- *upavistha konasana* (page 98), for 3–5 minutes;
- *savasana* (page 108), for 5 minutes.

Certain poses are best left out of a pregnancy routine, especially in the first trimester when there is a greater risk of miscarriage. These include abdominal exercises, strong twists and backbends.

As most new mothers will attest, motherhood is a work-out in itself. The constant bending, lifting and carrying all take their toll on the mother's body, which is still recovering from childbirth. Yoga is a perfect regime for mothers, because they can get back into exercising gently and progress gradually, and home practice fits in easily with the baby's nap time.

New mothers who take up yoga are usually very motivated to lose extra weight and tone flabby muscles. What they also discover is that the restorative poses and the yoga relaxation time recharge their batteries and lift their spirits. This way of exercising is a mood-enhancer for 'post-partum blues' and gives the mother renewed energy for the demands made on her by her infant. It's a matter of being rejuvenated each day, rather than feeling drained, as can sometimes happen.

For postnatal women, it is recommended not to do any yoga in the first six weeks after birth, apart from the yoga relaxation. Walking is good exercise, and the baby will enjoy some fresh air and a stroll, too. After that six-week period has elapsed, the new mother can gradually begin with the menstrual sequence and build up to standing poses, forward bends, twists and simple backbends as her stamina improves. Since the yoga postures help regulate the endocrine (hormonal) system, any postnatal depression may be relieved, and, in time, supplanted by a sense of calm. The habit of regular practice, cultivated over the preceding nine months, encourages the new mother to take care of herself, as well as the infant.

Menopause

This stage of woman's life is receiving more attention than ever before, as 'baby boomers' reach middle age. One estimate says that in the next 20 years, 40 million women will go through menopause in the United States alone!

The best approach to menopause is to think in terms of *prevention* of some symptoms. This is especially true given the increased longevity in the Western world: women will spend a third of their lives post-menopause.

Exercise can help prevent post-menopausal osteoporosis, and yoga is a particularly good remedy, as it works on the bones and joints, as well as on balancing the hormonal system. Regular yoga practice stimulates endorphin production and raises serotonin levels to help create a greater sense of wellbeing. The yoga relaxation offers an especially welcome respite from some of the emotional stresses that arise during this time of major changes.

My regular yoga practice over so many years has helped me gain a more detached attitude toward the ageing process that menopause heralds. Although our cultural conditioning says youth is everything, I know that wisdom comes with age, and contentment and self-awareness come with long-term yoga practice.

Breathing

The importance of working with the breath in yoga practice cannot be stressed strongly enough. While you don't have to learn complicated breathing techniques, you may have some bad breathing habits to unlearn.

One habit you'll need to break is suppressing the breath. Holding our breath is an ingrained behaviour that comes to the fore whenever we encounter a new and potentially stressful situation. As a beginner yoga student (and not even always as a beginner!), you will tend to hold your breath, because you are learning some unusual movements and exercising previously uncharted areas of your body. Holding your breath is extremely counterproductive, because when you hold your breath your muscles become tighter and tighter. This tension puts your nervous system on red alert, which then creates more stress and you lose any sensitivity to feeling what's going on in your body.

However, if you breathe quietly and evenly, you calm the nervous system and sensitise your body.

By reminding yourself to 'breathe through' resistance as it comes up, you'll be able to release any sign of tension straight away. In my experience, it takes time, patience and vigilance to correct this habit of holding the breath. It also takes a certain humility to remind yourself continually to check and see if you are, in fact, breathing. Don't just assume that you are.

The best way to use the breath in your poses is to follow the natural inclination to inhale when you're opening your chest and to exhale when you're compressing it. When you go into an expansive, chest-opening posture, such as stretching your arms overhead, you use a deep inhalation. When you bend your body forward or perform any contracting movement, you use a deep exhalation. When you are holding a pose, continue to breathe normally for as long as you are in the pose.

Here's how it works, for example, when moving from *tadasana*, the basic standing pose (page 78), to *uttanasana*, the standing forward bend (page 72). (You may want to stop reading for a moment and try out this sequence of movements to get the hang of it.) First, you stand upright, breathing naturally. When you're ready to move, stretch the arms up, inhaling deeply. Then, bend forward, exhaling deeply. Hold the pose for a few normal breaths and, when you're ready to come up again, begin inhaling as you stretch the arms up, and let the torso follow. When you're upright again, exhale steadily and bring the arms back down.

You may have noticed when doing this sequence that when you inhaled fully, the lungs opened up, and when you exhaled fully, the muscles soften and you could perhaps stretch out a little more.

It's a good idea to time yourself in a pose by using your breath instead of the clock. By counting breaths rather than minutes, you will also be observing the quality of the breath, checking to see that you're not labouring at it or holding it.

Early on in your yoga practice, it will seem like you have no idea how to coordinate your body and your breath, or how to focus your awareness internally. Don't worry, it just takes time. Every time you repeat a pose, you are creating new links between your brain and your muscles, and the more you practise, the deeper these links will become.

Another poor breathing habit is tightening the diaphragm, the muscle at the bottom of the rib cage which internally divides the chest from the abdomen. Some of us have learned to tense our diaphragm unconsciously through emotional trauma or through trying to 'improve' our posture by sticking our chests out and sucking our bellies in.

Having a hard, flat stomach is not conducive to breathing easily, and only when you relax your chest and abdomen is your diaphragm able to do it's job well. Diaphragmatic breathing is a more efficient way to breathe than upper-chest or thoracic breathing. It's done by releasing the abdomen and diaphragm (breathing in) and contracting them (breathing out). Some people abhor the look and thought of their stomach protruding, as it does when it's relaxed and released with the inhalation. However, the way you exercise and your normal posture should give your stomach muscles and internal organs tone, not chronic contraction. Just watch how naturally a baby breathes, with its abdomen and diaphragm completely soft.

As adults, we need to find our way back to that naturalness of the baby, by being attentive to our body and our breath. This way, yoga poses feel natural and unforced. I remind my students that the breath is everything. It's our very life force.

Yoga poses involve straightforward movements, yet it takes intentional awareness to ensure the poses are never done in a perfunctory or unconscious manner. Monitoring the breath helps keep us from working mechanically in the poses.

I've found listening to my breath as I practise yoga to be a very effective focal point. I deliberately turn up the volume on the sound of my breath, so I can hear it more easily. This is called *ujjayi* breathing, where you draw the breath in and out from the back of the throat. I can adjust my breath in this way so that it has a calm sound, like a lullaby, or a powerful sound, like bellows stoking a fire. Modulating your breath in this way is helpful when you want to still or clear your mind, when you want help falling asleep, when you need to focus and when you want to release tension.

The breath acts as a bridge between our psyche and our physique in yoga practice, just as it does in many other situations in our lives. It could be called the 'psycho-physiological' aspect, the interface of mind and body. This is one of the aspects of yoga that has kept me so interested over the years.

I first observed this link many years ago, when watching a friend doing her yoga postures with a grace that seemed unavailable to me at the time. She performed the poses with what is sometimes referred to as 'effortless effort'. She worked deeply in the poses, but never appeared to be trying so hard that she had difficulty breathing. On the contrary, to get deeper into a pose, she would use her breath as a vehicle. As she exhaled, she could lengthen more into a stretch because she was letting go of resistance. I realised that because she wasn't tensing, her muscles were more relaxed.

When you learn to coordinate yoga stretching with smooth, steady inhalations and exhalations, you can both soften in a pose and hold it for extended periods. Breathing gets you through what, for novices, can be the initial discomfort of training your muscles and bones to move in completely new ways. If you try too hard to achieve a pose, the body seizes up and stubbornly resists any further opening up. The muscles baulk at the stress and, given time, the cells of the body become depleted from the sustained effort. Frustration arises, as well as impatience! The mind yells, 'I'm outta here!', and you find yourself out of the pose before you know what happened. Instead of being so reactive, keep coming back to deepening your breath. You'll open up in the pose and have a fuller sense of who you are.

Once you learn to let your breath flow consistently and steadily, which *does* take time, attention and repetition, your practice will become very satisfying indeed. It's not that you are applying yourself any less, but because you are being led by your breath, you are much more in the moment. The practice flows.

Putting it all together

Some students are very keen and absolutely love yoga, but only ever come to classes and don't do their own practice. They know they ought to, but they don't. One reason for this is that they feel overwhelmed about where to begin. Fair enough. One well-subscribed yoga book has over 200 poses in it, and these have been distilled from thousands of poses, including all the yoga variations and preparations. What beginner wouldn't feel lost deciding what and how to practise!

In your practice, you may find it helpful to remember the advice given by the King in *Alice in Wonderland*: 'Begin at the beginning...and go on till you come to the end; then stop'. The order in which you do the poses is totally logical. Every practice has a beginning, a middle and an end. First, you warm up your body, then you challenge yourself with more dynamic poses, and, finally, you slow down and soothe your body.

One advantage of practising in this methodical way is that it is easier for you to assess the effects that each pose and specific sequence of poses has on you.

Keep it simple. Start by practising only a few poses. Gradually add more postures to your repertoire once you've worked with the original ones for some time.

The middle section of any practice period for beginners should be the standing poses, because they help cultivate strength and suppleness, energy, relaxation and focus.

In the beginning, your poses may not look picture-perfect, like the photographs you see presented in this book. The yogis in these pictures have trained their bodies over many years. Remember, yoga practice is a *process*, and forcing poses before your body is ready to open up can impede your progress.

Brief practices

Short practices on a regular basis are infinitely better in terms of your yoga progress than a once-a-week marathon session. This is why people who come to one yoga class a week (or less frequently) get less out of their yoga than those who practice at home as well. If you're limited by your schedule, do what you can, even if it's a little every day, because you'll find that as you start to feel the benefits, you will make more time for yoga.

A succinct but energetic practice is to do *surya namaskar* (salutes to the sun — page 76) for 15 minutes first thing in the morning. This helps to charge up your body, because the breathing is strong and rhythmical. And even doing such a short practice warrants a 5-minute *savasana* (relaxation).

Another short practice you could try includes a variety of the standing poses: *tadasana, urdhva hastasana, trikonasana, virabhadrasana II, parsvakonasana, parsvottanasana* and *prasarita padottanasana* (pages 78–88). Do them in sequence repeating two or three times for 15 minutes, followed by *savasana* (page 108).

If you are menstruating or feel tired, a good mini-sequence is *Supta baddha konasana* (page 105), *upavistha konasana* (supine splits with the legs on the wall — page 99), and legs-on-a-chair *viparita karani* (page 106), held for 5 minutes each, followed by *savasana* (page 108).

Once you get the hang of balancing a sequence of postures, you can make up your own short sequences that incorporate all of the following four phases: centring, warm-up, dynamic and cool-down.

Centring yourself

A gentle way to ease into your practice is to do *supta baddha konasana* (page 105). Centring time is essential for you to mentally and physically arrive in your body if you have been busy beforehand. Because you are quiet in the pose, it gives you a chance to 'check in' with your body to determine your energy level. You are able to assess whether you have any particular physical or emotional needs to address in the practice. You may find that it is more appropriate to do restorative poses, for example, or that you really need to increase your energy with dynamic poses. Be sensitive to how your body and mind are feeling, as this changes according to diet, weather and your mood. Be aware of what your attitude reflects as you approach your practice, and respect your limits.

Starting with *supta baddha konasana* (page 105) is a great way to settle your mind. Even if you're doing an early morning practice and you haven't been awake for long, it's quite amazing how the mind can generate hundreds of things to do and places to go. *Supta baddha konasana* helps give the groin a good stretch, too, and opens up the chest, abdomen and pelvis.

When you've completed *supta baddha konasana* and you sit up again, simply bend forward in the kneeling position, *virasana* forward stretch (page 95), for a minute or so, to stretch your shoulders.

Gradual stretching is the key to warming up and is essential to avoid injuring muscles. It helps create optimum joint movement and ensures that the joints are lubricated and unrestricted right from the start of your practice.

Warming up

Good warm-up poses to do are: *adho mukha svanasana* (downward-facing dog pose — page 71), *uttanasana* (standing forward bend — page 72) and the *supta padangusthasana* cycle (the lying-down leg stretches — page 73).

The right-angle stretch (page 68) and the chest-opener and

shoulder stretch (page 69) are perfect for loosening muscle tension in the upper body as you prepare to take on more intense postures. *Adho mukha svanasana* helps stretch the backs of the legs. Repeat it several times with *uttanasana* or *virasana* forward stretch in between to slowly increase the stretch to your leg muscles and spinal column. Lunges work well in this phase, as do *surya namaskar* (salutes to the sun — page 76), if they are done slowly, emphasising *ujjayi* breathing.

Dynamic, intense phase

The importance of doing the more intense poses is to improve your flexibility and circulation, to breathe more deeply and to increase stamina and strength. As you work more strongly in this phase, all the various systems of the body are affected, including nervous, glandular, eliminative and digestive systems.

Standing poses should be included in every practice, especially when you are a beginner, because they are readily achieved and provide many benefits. I call them 'gatekeeper' poses, because they safely provide the joint and muscle flexibility and stamina that will later allow you to adopt more advanced poses with relative ease and little danger of injury.

After several *adho mukha svanasana* (downward-facing dog) poses, do a couple of the standing poses, each one done once to each side, and then repeated two or three times, to help you begin to understand them better. This will also help develop your focus. Doing repetitions of the poses deepens the connection between the brain and the various parts of the body, and you start to get more of a sense of the flow and movement of the practice.

It is during this more intense phase that you might want to include *surya namaskar* poses (salutes to the sun), and begin to do them more quickly. To create a more intense work-out, you can include a standing pose (between the downward-facing dog poses) in the middle of each of the salutes. Abdominal exercises are included in the dynamic phase, too.

If you wish to do some backbends in this section, be sure to follow them with a twist performed two or three times, as a counter pose. Twists are beneficial if your back is sore. For beginners, *ardha jathara parivartanasana* (lying-down twist — page 103) works best.

Forward bends are a good transition into the quietening phase, particularly when you do them for shorter timings, then repeat them for a slightly longer timing. For example, you could do *janu sirsasana* (head-to-knee pose — page 96) holding for 1 minute each side, repeat, and then do it one more time for 2 minutes on each side. This has the effect of cooling down and sedating the brain, especially if you rest your forehead on a bolster or the seat of a chair.

Quietening down

In the quietening-down phase at the end of your practice, it is good to include a lying-down pose such as *supta baddha konasana* (page 105), which you hold for 5 minutes, keeping your eyes covered. *Viparita karani* (legs-up-the-wall or on a chair — page 106) is also an important resting pose, partly because it lets gravity do the work while you let go completely. It takes no energy from you, but gives energy back by soothing the nervous system and settling the body and mind.

The resting poses and relaxation alleviate any shakiness you may experience after the active poses, and also eliminate the 'wired-up' feeling that can sometimes result from doing a strong work-out.

Your aim is to feel vital and fit after yoga. You will routinely complete your practice with the yoga relaxation, to help 'centre' yourself and to get in touch with your own inner light.

5 THE POSTURES

Sitting poses

The following poses help warm up the ligaments, tendons and muscles of the shoulders, knees, ankles, feet and hips, as all those joints are moved in various ways.

Unless you are flexible, you will need to sit on a folded blanket or cushion to keep your spine straighter and provide more comfort.

VIRASANA

HERO'S POSE

Virasana *relieves stiffness in the knees, ankles and quadriceps (front thigh muscles). It is a particularly good pose for people who regularly stand for hours on end. Buddhist monks often adopt this posture during long periods of meditation because it helps them to keep the spine upright. You can do virasana in your practice after the standing poses, to rest the leg muscles.*

Equipment: blanket (optional).

Kneel down, spread your feet apart, keeping your knees together, and sit between your heels.

If there is pressure on your knees or ankle joints, or your buttocks don't touch the floor, sit on a folded blanket so that your buttocks are fully supported.

Place your palms on the soles of your feet, your fingers on your toes.

Stretch your trunk upwards and bring your shoulders down while sitting with your spine erect.

Breathe normally. Stay in the pose for I minute at first, gradually building up to 5 minutes as you become more experienced.

To release the pose, place your hands on the floor next to your hips and stretch your legs out in front of you.

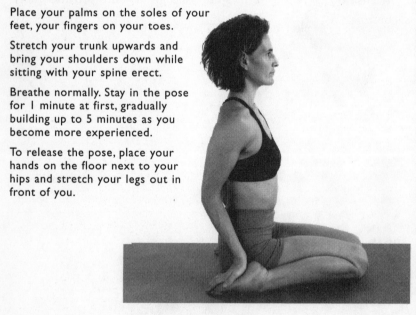

SUKHASANA
EASY CROSS-LEGGED POSE

This pose is also called the 'tailor's pose', as it is the seated posture adopted by tailors in India. It is the simplest of seated meditation poses, allowing the meditator to sit firmly upright, yet still be relaxed. Sukhasana is good for loosening hips, knees and ankles, and strengthening the back.

Equipment: blanket.

Sit on a folded blanket and fold your legs into a loose cross-legged position.

Press your fingertips down on the floor on either side of your hips and lift your trunk up straight.

Variation I: Keeping your spine straight, release your hands, bring them onto your lap and interlock your fingers. Turn your palms outwards and extend your arms up over your head. Firm your elbows so that your arms are completely straight.

Keep extending your arms and trunk upwards, and bring your shoulders and shoulder blades down.

Breathing normally, hold the pose for about 30 seconds.

Bring your arms down and release your hands.

Reverse the way you crossed your legs and reverse the way you interlocked your fingers, so that the other thumb is on top. Repeat the arm stretch and hold for 30 seconds. Release your arms and hands, and stretch out your legs.

Variation 2: To stretch your back more in *sukhasana*, place your hands onto the floor in front of you and stretch forwards. As long as you can keep extending your back straight, take your chest and forehead nearer to the floor.

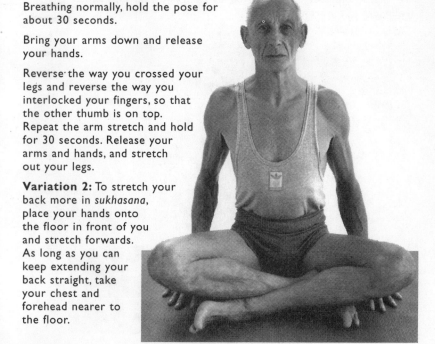

BADDHA KONASANA

BOUND-ANGLE POSE

This pose is nicknamed 'cobbler's pose', and I have actually seen Indian shoemakers sitting in this position as they work. Baddha konasana helps loosen tight groins and hips.

Equipment: blanket (optional).

Sit on the floor with your legs straight out in front of you. If your back muscles are very tight, you can do this pose seated on the edge of a folded blanket or with your back against a wall for support.

Bend your knees to the sides and bring the soles of your feet together, pulling your heels in as close to the pubis as possible.

Clasp your hands around your feet, and, as you pull on your feet, stretch your spine upwards. Open and lift your chest.

Avoid rounding your back and keep your shoulders down.

Breathe normally. Hold the pose for 1–2 minutes, stretching your knees towards the floor.

To release the pose, bring your hands alongside your hips and stretch your legs out in front of you.

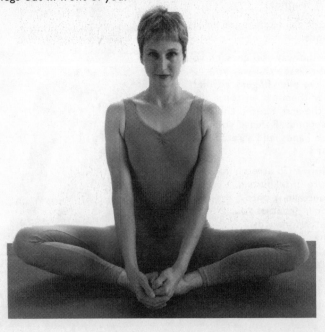

Variation: To further stretch the groin, stretch your trunk forwards, with your elbows pressing against the inside of your thighs. As long as you can keep your spine extended, take your chest and forehead nearer to the floor.

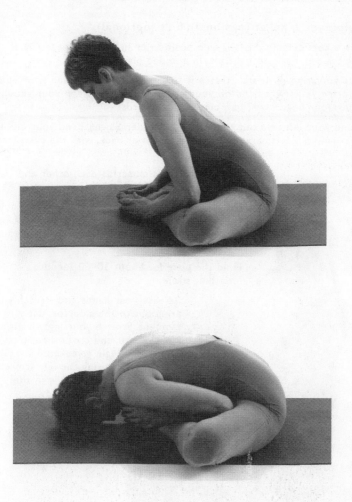

GOMUKHASANA

COW'S HEAD POSE

Gomukhasana is so named because the positioning of the arms (supposedly) forms the shape of a cow's horns ... In any case, this one of the best poses for loosening up upper-back tightness and facilitating shoulder-joint flexibility. It is a satisfying pose for everyday practice, because you can see yourself progress quickly and your shoulders feel so good afterwards.

Equipment: blanket (optional); belt (optional).

Sit in a comfortable cross-legged position or in *virasana* (page 62). If your back or hips are tight, sit on a folded blanket.

Raise your right arm and stretch it towards the ceiling. Bend your elbow and place your right hand on your upper back, in between your shoulder blades. Your fingers will be pointing downwards.

Extend your left arm out sideways at shoulder height, bend your elbow and place your left hand in the middle of your back, with the palm facing out.

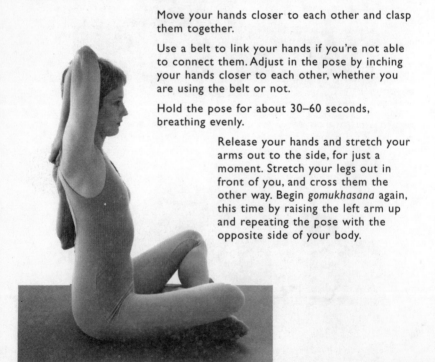

Move your hands closer to each other and clasp them together.

Use a belt to link your hands if you're not able to connect them. Adjust in the pose by inching your hands closer to each other, whether you are using the belt or not.

Hold the pose for about 30–60 seconds, breathing evenly.

Release your hands and stretch your arms out to the side, for just a moment. Stretch your legs out in front of you, and cross them the other way. Begin *gomukhasana* again, this time by raising the left arm up and repeating the pose with the opposite side of your body.

PARIPURNA NAVASANA

FULL BOAT POSE

This pose is excellent for toning abdominal muscles and is a good remedy for digestive problems and flatulence, because the internal organs are stimulated. It also helps develop concentration and focus. If you have pain in your back, or if you are menstruating or pregnant, do not practice this pose.

Sit on the floor with your legs stretched straight in front of you and pressed together.

Place your hands on the floor next to your hips.

Bend your legs in towards your chest, lean back slightly, then raise your legs, and re-straighten them.

Extend your arms forwards until they are parallel with the floor, with the palms facing each other.

Keep your knees and elbows locked.

Lift your chest; your big toes should be in line with your eyes.

Hold the pose for 20–30 seconds. There is a tendency to hold the breath, so be aware of your breathing and breathe evenly throughout.

Bend your legs, place your feet on the floor and lie on your back.

Variation: If your abdominal muscles are weak, your back muscles are probably weak too, so you may want to practise this pose with the soles of your feet on the wall, in line with your head. Alternatively, you can hold the backs of your thighs when your legs are raised.

Repeat this pose two or three times, gradually building up the repetitions and increasing the length of time you hold the pose.

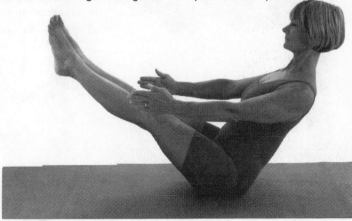

Warm-up poses

RIGHT-ANGLE STRETCH

Although not a classic yoga pose, the right-angle stretch is one of the most effective techniques for the relief of back tension ever conceived. It restores elasticity to the back muscles and is especially useful after hours of pouring over books and/or sitting at a computer. If you have trouble with adho mukha svanasana *(downward-facing dog pose) on page 71, doing the right-angle stretch first for a short period will help you warm up for it.*

Stand in front of a wall and place your hands on the wall in line with your hips. Your hands should be shoulder-width distance apart and in one line.

Keeping your hands firmly on the wall, walk slowly backwards, bending forwards, until your arms are straight and your torso is parallel with the floor.

Keep your feet hip-width distance apart and parallel, and your legs straight.

Don't let your back sway. Keep your navel drawing upwards.

If you notice that your back is rounding or that your shoulders feel tense, take your hands a little higher up the wall.

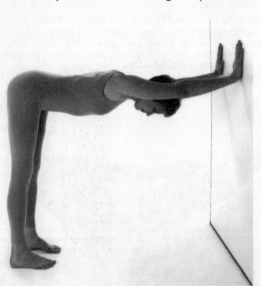

As you press your hands in to the wall, move your buttocks towards the centre of the room, to create a cross-tension stretch.

Hold the position for 1–2 minutes, breathing evenly, then walk in a step or two as you inhale and come up.

CHEST-OPENER AND SHOULDER STRETCH

Again, this is not an authentic yoga pose, but is particularly valuable for those of you who spend a lot of time hunched over a computer keyboard. This pose can be repeated often throughout the day, whenever you notice your shoulders are feeling tense.

Position yourself in front of a window ledge or a high bench.

Bend your arms and place your elbows on the edge of the ledge. Press the palms of your hands together over your head. Keep your elbows shoulder-width distance apart.

Walk slowly backwards, until your back is straight and parallel with the floor and your legs are at a right-angle to your trunk.

If you are quite supple, bring your elbows closer together; if your shoulders and/or back is stiff, move your elbows further apart.

Check that your feet are hip-width distance apart, your legs are straight, and your spine and shoulders are stretching away from your head.

Hold the pose for 1–2 minutes, breathing evenly.

Release your hands, walk in a step or two and inhale as you come up.

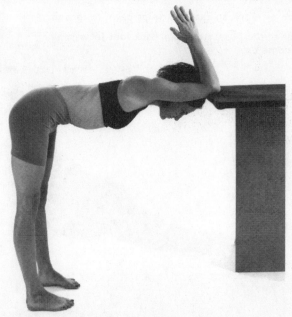

LUNGE

This pose is good for hip flexibility. It stretches the front thigh muscles and helps the knee and ankle joints.

Equipment: 2 blocks (optional).

Kneel down in an all-fours position and step your right foot forward between your hands. Your right leg is now in a lunge position and your left knee is on the floor.

Rest your fingertips on the floor so that your hands are shaped like a dome. (Your hands can be supported on blocks if you find it difficult to reach the floor.)

Ensure your hips are squarely facing forwards and your right buttock is moving downwards. Lift your chest up towards the ceiling.

If there is no strain, tighten your left knee and work on straightening your left leg. Push your left heel further back.

Continue to keep your shoulders down and your chest up. Avoid arching your neck backwards, especially if it is tight.

Hold the pose for 4 or 5 long breaths, then reverse the legs and repeat all of the above adjustments on the second side.

Repeat twice or more, so that your hips begin to loosen.

To come out of the pose, step your back foot forward and slowly come up.

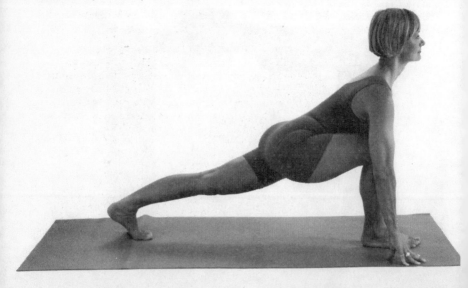

ADHO MUKHA SVANASANA

DOWNWARD-FACING DOG POSE

This pose stretches the shoulders, back muscles and spine to help relieve fatigue. It also stretches the backs of the legs and the Achilles tendons.

Equipment: blanket or bolster or block (optional; see note).

Kneel down in an all-fours position. Place your hands shoulder-width distance apart and position them right underneath your shoulders. Place your feet hip-width distance apart.

Stretch the palms of your hands, spreading your fingers, and make sure the middle finger is pointing straight ahead.

Tuck your toes under, raise your buttocks and straighten your arms and legs.

Your body should now be in an inverted 'V' position, much the same as that of a dog when it's stretching after a sleep.

Release your shoulders by moving them away from your ears, back towards your hips. Relax the muscles in your neck and let your head hang down loosely.

Lift your hips a little higher, tighten your kneecaps and front thigh muscles.

Press the front of your leg towards the back of your leg and bring your heels closer to the floor, but continue to lift your hips and the back of your thighs upwards.

Hold the position for 30–60 seconds, breathing evenly, then exhale and kneel back down to rest.

Note: You can rest your head on a folded blanket, bolster or block to make this a more restful pose or to hold it for a longer period of time. Even with your head supported, keep your arms and legs straight.

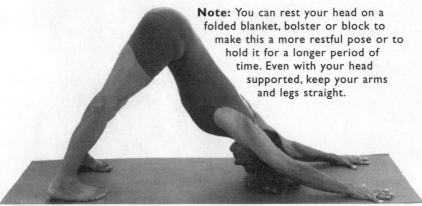

UTTANASANA

STANDING FORWARD BEND

Uttanasana is a particularly effective stretch for the back muscles and legs. Because you are in an inverted position with your head down, the brain is quietened, especially if this pose is done with your head supported on the seat of a chair or a bolster. If you are very stiff or feel any discomfort when bending forward, keep your knees flexed.

Stand with your feet hip-width distance apart, inhale and stretch your arms straight up over your head, and bend forwards from your hips.

Keep your kneecaps pulled up, exhale and extend your trunk and your arms down. Roll your shoulders out.

Relax your neck and let your head hang loosely. Keep breathing evenly.

If your body is stiff and your back is tending to bow, hold on to your shins and keep your chest lifted a little. Those of you who are more supple can place your hands on the floor beside your feet.

Keep your shoulders pulled up towards your waist, even as you stretch your trunk down. Your abdomen is drawn back towards your back bone.

Hold the pose for 30–60 seconds. With each exhalation, soften your back muscles, but keep your legs firm.

Bend your knees slightly and inhale as you come up.

Variation: For a more restorative pose, rest your buttocks on a wall, with your feet about 20 cm away from the wall and your head and arms supported on the seat of a chair. Stay in this position for 2 or 3 minutes.

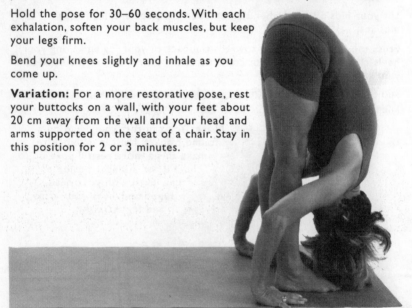

SUPTA PADANGUSTHASANA
LYING-DOWN LEG STRETCHES — THREE VARIATIONS

This sequence is simply the best for stretching hamstrings and improving hip flexibility. I also recommend it for some sciatica problems.

Equipment: belt; blanket.

Variation 1: Lie down near to a wall with your back on the floor and your head supported on a folded blanket. Keep your legs and feet together and straight, and the soles of your feet flush against the wall.

Bend your right leg in towards the outer-right chest, and, using both hands, hug your leg to your chest. Don't let your left foot come away from the wall.

Keep your left leg straight, with the back of your thigh and knee on the floor.

Hold the pose for 10–15 long breaths, then either release the pose, or continue into Variation 2.

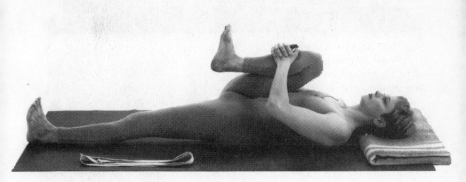

Variation 2: Remain in the Variation 1 pose, then slip the belt over the ball of your right foot and straighten your right leg towards the ceiling. Keep both hands holding onto each side of the belt.

Keep your chest open and your shoulders and throat relaxed.

Stay in position for about 10–15 breaths and work on extending both your legs, breathing evenly. Release the pose or continue into Variation 3.

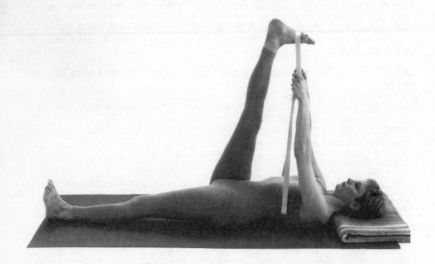

Variation 3: With your right leg still raised, hold the belt in the right hand and extend your left arm onto the floor on the left side, palm upwards, in line with your left shoulder.

Keep your left foot pressing on the wall, your left leg straight and your left hip on the floor. Keep turning your left thigh inwards.

Slowly take your right leg out to the right side, in line with the right hip, as far as your flexibility will allow. It is better to keep your leg straight than to bend it and go all the way to the floor.

To avoid rolling your trunk over to the right, keep your navel turning to the left. Your chest should also be turning to the left as you take your right leg further to the right, and your left buttock should stay firmly on the floor.

Hold this extension for about 10–15 breaths.

Bring your right leg back up to a vertical position, exhale, and lower it to the floor alongside your left leg.

Bring your legs back together, and check that the soles of both feet are touching the wall again.

Repeat all the three variations with the left leg.

The length of time you stay in the pose can be gradually extended in Variations 2 and 3. I've reached the stage where I can hold them for 5 minutes each side, but that has taken me many years.

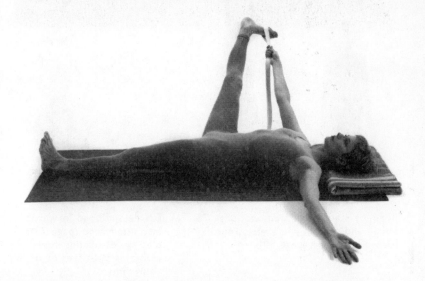

SURYA NAMASKAR

SALUTE TO THE SUN

Surya namaskar *(salute to the sun)* is so named because it was usually executed before sunrise. This sequence incorporates several of the preceding poses. It is a simple and efficient way to practise if you have limited time, because it takes your body through a range of stretching, strengthening and joint-rotating exercises in a relatively short period of time. Ten or 15 minutes of 'salutes' is guaranteed to get your heart going and blow away any cobwebs.

It is best to start this sequence slowly and to warm up gradually. Proceeding slowly also helps you to take all the time you need to execute each separate movement more precisely and to get into the proper alignment. Then, after a few rounds, as your breathing increases, you will naturally want to accelerate the speed of your movements.

The flow of surya namaskar is like a choreographed dance, so it may take you a few repetitions to remember the sequence. Once you've mastered that, you'll be able to move smoothly and rhythmically from one pose to the next. The breath is what facilitates smooth transitions, so be sure to follow the prescribed breathing instructions.

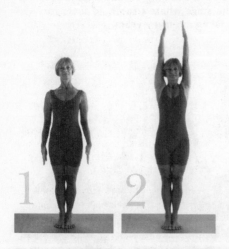 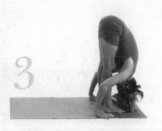

Begin by standing in *tadasana* (page 78). Inhale and stretch you arms up into *urdhva hastasana* (page 80).

Exhale and bend forwards into *uttanasana* (page 72), placing your hands down alongside your feet or on your shins.

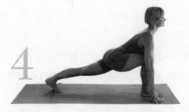

4

Bend your knees, place your hands on the floor on either side of your right foot, inhale and step your left foot back to a lunge position (page 70).

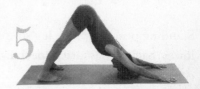

5

Exhale and step your right foot back, parallel with the left, for *adho mukha svanasana* (page 71). Hold the pose for 5 breaths.

6

Inhale and step your left foot forwards to the lunge position.

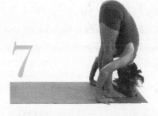

7

Exhale, step your right foot forwards, alongside the left, bending forwards in *uttanasana* again, with your hands on the floor or on your shins.

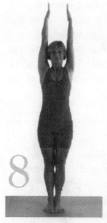

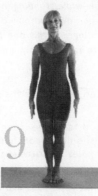

8

Inhale and raise your arms overhead for *urdhva hastasana*.

9

Exhale as you lower your arms.

Before starting the next round, check that your feet are back together and that you're standing in *tadasana*.

Repeat the sequence as above, this time stepping your right foot back in a lunge position.

Beginners can do two or three rounds of the sequence, gradually building up to 10 rounds.

Standing poses

Standing poses improve leg strength and flexibility of the hips and lower back. They are especially good for creating a feeling of centredness and stability.

Keep watching to see what your weak areas are, for example, tight groins. Working on your weak areas, perhaps doing several repetitions of the same pose, until you begin to see changes occurring.

Note: For standing poses it helps to be on a non-skid mat, especially if you're working on a slippery surface.

TADASANA

MOUNTAIN POSE

This is the basic pose, because it teaches you to have excellent posture while standing, which is then hopefully reproduced whenever you're walking or sitting. You can practise this pose surreptitiously while standing in a queue at the bank or the bus stop. Some yoga students who have had only a few lessons say that their posture improves from understanding just this one pose. From tadasana, we learn balance and symmetry and to re-adjust our posture in many of the other poses.

Stand straight with your feet together and your arms gently stretched by the side of your body.

The placement of your feet is all-important. The inner arches of your feet and the inside of your big toes should be touching, and your weight should be evenly distributed on the soles of both feet.

Lift and stretch all your toes, then bring them back into contact with the floor, still extended. (You may find that your toes are stiff and don't respond, in which case you can bend over and manually move them apart to give them more of a stretch.)

Press the base of your big toes and the inside heels into the floor, and draw up the inner ankle bones. Keep the arches of your feet lifted.

Pull up your kneecaps up and tighten your front thigh muscles (quadriceps).

Roll your thighs in and move your tail-bone downwards. Move your front thighbones back. Squeeze in your outer hips.

Stretch your spine up, including the back of your neck. Lift your breastbone and back ribs, but not your shoulders. Move your shoulders down and your shoulder blades inwards.

Move the crown of your head towards the ceiling. Your head should be straight, your chin level with the ground and your ears in line with your shoulders. Relax your face completely, keeping your eyes soft and looking straight ahead.

Stay in the pose for 30–60 seconds, breathing evenly.

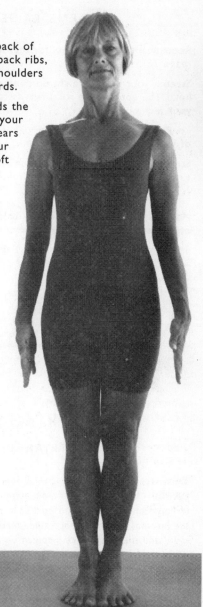

URDHVA HASTASANA

ARMS-RAISED TADASANA

Repeat all the adjustments for *tadasana* (page 78).

Stretch your arms straight up over your head. The upper arms roll inwards towards your face.

Lock your elbows in, with the palms of your hands facing each other.

Stretch up the both sides of your body evenly, without hunching your shoulders.

Move your shoulder blades in.

Make sure your weight is evenly balanced on the soles of both feet.

Stay in the pose for 30 seconds. Exhale and bring your arms down by the sides of your body.

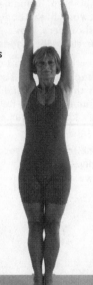

TRIKONASANA

TRIANGLE POSTURE

Trikonasana benefits feet, ankles and legs, and gives a strong lateral stretch. Because side-stretching movements are uncommon in day-to-day life, trikonasana can help with backache and neck stiffness, and it also massages the internal organs on each side, particularly the liver and gall bladder on the right, and the stomach and spleen on the left.

Beginners sometimes have difficulty keeping their arms raised continuously. If so, before you repeat the pose on the left side, rest your hands on your hips. However, if you can manage to keep your arms elevated, it will help you develop greater upper body strength.

Stand in *tadasana* (page 78). Step your feet your own leg-length apart. Turn your left foot in about 20 degrees and your right foot out exactly 90 degrees.

Check that the heel of your right foot is in a direct line with the arch of your left foot.

Extend your arms out level with your shoulders.

Flex your right thigh and check to make sure that your right knee is pointing in the same direction as your right foot.

Stretch your right arm out further to the right, then bend sideways to the right, keeping your head, arms, shoulders and hips squared, facing the same direction.

Place your right hand down on your right shin, near to your knee, and stretch your left arm up to the ceiling. The left palm faces the same way as the front of your body.

Pull up your knees and front thigh muscles. Tuck your right butock in and take your left hip up and back.

If you find that you can turn your neck easily, look up at your left hand; if not, look forward.

Extend the back of your neck away from your shoulders and move your shoulders down towards your waist.

Hold the pose for 10–15 breaths, then inhale, coming up with the arms still outstretched.

Reverse the position of your feet, and repeat the position on the left side.

Step back to *tadasana*.

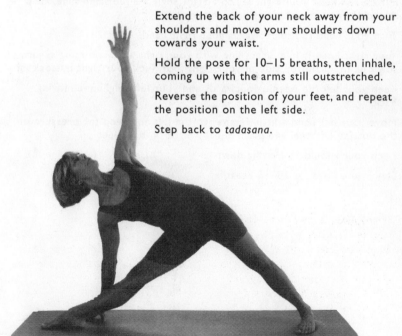

VIRABHADRASANA II

WARRIOR POSE

This pose reflects the energy of a warrior, with qualities of strength, centredness and vigilance. Virabhadrasana II is effective in strengthening the legs, stretching the groin and improving hip flexibility.

Stand in *tadasana* (page 78). Step your feet a little wider than your leg-width apart.

Extend your arms sideways level with your shoulders, palms facing down.

Your whole body should be squarely facing forward: head, arms, shoulders, hips and legs.

Turn both your feet to the right; your left foot only slightly and your right foot 90 degrees. The heel of your right foot should be in line with the inner arch of your left foot.

Pull up your knees and front thigh muscles.

Exhale and bend your right leg to a right angle. At the same time, keep stretching and straightening your left leg.

Turn your head to look towards your right hand.

Your right knee is in a direct line with your right ankle, pointing slightly towards the little-toe side of your right foot. Tuck your right buttock in.

Keep your left hip opening outwards and your left thighbone moving back.

Move your left hand a little further to the left and keep the pressure on the outside left heel and place equal weight on both feet.

Keep your shoulders moving down.

Stay in the pose for 10–15 breaths.

Inhale as you straighten your right leg and turn both feet to the left side.

If your arms get tired, place your hands on your hips while you're turning your feet, and then re-stretch them.

Repeat the sequence of adjustments on the left side.

Turn your feet to face the front, and step back to *tadasana*.

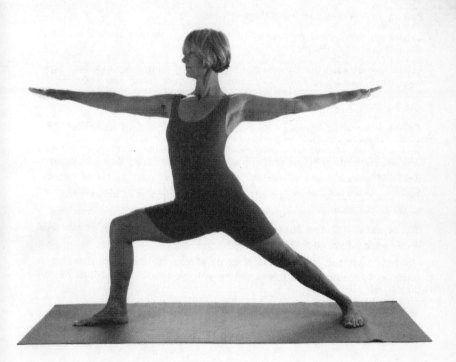

PARSVAKONASANA
SIDE-ANGLE POSE

This pose tones the leg muscles and helps generate and build up stamina.

Equipment: block (optional).

Stand in *tadasana* (page 78). Step your feet a little wider than leg-length apart. Extend the arms sideways, parallel with the floor.

Turn your right foot out 90 degrees and your left foot slightly in.

Pull up your knees and front thigh muscles.

Exhale and bend your right knee to a right angle. At the same time, keep the left leg very straight.

Exhale and stretch the ribs on the right side of your body out over your right thigh, and place your right hand on the outside of your right foot. (If you experience any difficulty reaching the floor, place your hand on a block on the outside of your right foot.)

Keep moving your left thigh back and rolling your left hip upwards.

Take your left arm up over your head, with the biceps over your left ear, and stretch your arm out straight with your palm facing down towards the floor.

Turn the right side of your waist forwards and turn your breastbone towards the ceiling.

If your neck is able to rotate freely, turn your head and look up towards the ceiling; if not, look straight ahead.

Hold the pose for 10–15 breaths. Inhale as you come up, straightening your right leg. Reverse the feet and repeat the sequence of adjustments on the left side.

Turn your feet to face the front and step back to *tadasana*.

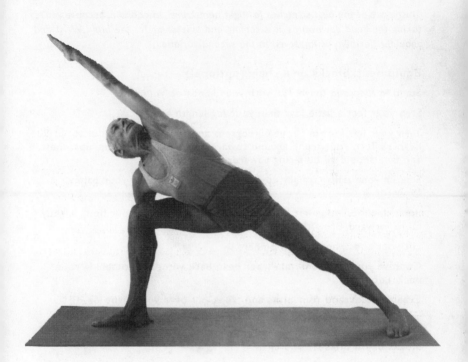

PARSVOTTANASANA

SIDEWAYS EXTENSION

This is one of the best stretches for tight hamstrings. In addition, because you're taking the head downwards, it is cooling and quietening for the brain. Wrist and shoulder flexibility is improved in the second variation.

Equipment: blocks or a chair (optional).

Stand in *tadasana* (page 78), with your hands on your hips.

Step your feet a little less than your leg-length apart.

Turn your left foot in about 60 degrees and your right foot out about 90 degrees. Turn your trunk around towards your right leg. Your hips, chest, and face should all be facing towards the right.

Stretch your arms straight up over your head, and turn your palms forwards.

Press down on your left heel and turn the left side of your body slightly more forward. Bring the right side slightly back.

Lift your chest, not your shoulders.

Concave your back and take your head back without shortening your neck. Look up.

Exhale and extend your arms and trunk out over your right leg.

Take your hands down and rest your fingertips on the floor on either side of your right foot. If your hands don't reach the floor, place them on blocks or on the seat of a chair.

Turn the left side of your body slightly to the right and bring right buttock slightly back. Both sides of the chest are equidistant from the floor.

Keep the knees firmly pulled up.

Breathe in deeply several times, relaxing your neck and letting your head hang loosely. Inhale and come up, stretching the arms up and then lowering them back down.

Reverse the position of your feet and repeat the above steps on the left side.

Turn your feet to face the front and step back to *tadasana*.

Variation: To provide more of a shoulder stretch and rotation, you can repeat this pose with your hands placed in 'prayer' position on your back, with your fingers pressed together between your shoulder blades, if possible (see photograph). When you finish the pose, release your arms and stretch them strongly out to the sides before lowering them.

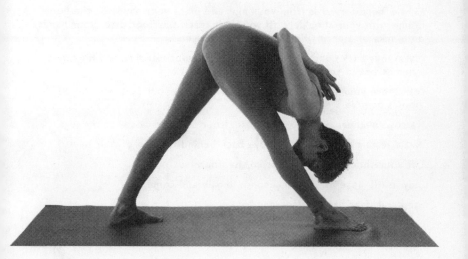

PRASARITA PADOTTANASANA

INTENSE FORWARD STRETCH

This pose is particularly good for stretching hamstrings, adductor muscles, and the spine. Prasarita padottanasana increases blood circulation to the head and upper body, because you're stretching your torso downwards.

Equipment: blocks or a chair (optional).

Stand in *tadasana* (page 78). Step your feet wide apart, somewhat wider than the other standing poses. Your feet should be parallel.

Place your hands on your hips, with your fingers pointing forwards.

Tighten your knees, lift your chest, inhale and look up.

Exhale, bend forwards from your hips and place your hands on the floor in line with your shoulders. (If you can't reach the floor, place your hands on blocks or a chair.) Keep your arms straight.

Make your back concave and look up. Keep your legs firm and lift the inner arches of your feet.

Next, take your hands further back, in line with your feet, with the elbows bent to a right angle.

Keep your knees pulled up, and bring your trunk in closer to the legs.

Avoid letting your buttocks move back behind the line of your heels.

Lift your shoulders up away from the floor.

Stay in the pose for 20–30 seconds. Inhale and come up.

Step your feet back to *tadasana*.

Variations:

1 Interlock your hands behind your back and stretch your arms straight up as you bend forwards.

2 Rest your forehead on a block or the seat of a chair (depending on your flexibility) when you're fully in the down position, and stay in the pose for 1–2 minutes.

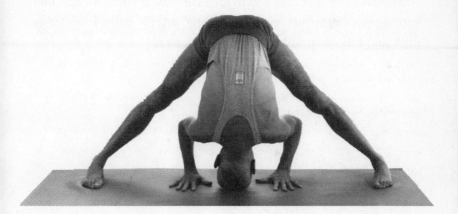

Backbends

Backbends stimulate the nervous system, open up the chest and correct stooped shoulders. They can help people who suffer from asthma, and are excellent for alleviating depression or even dispelling a case of the doldrums.

Backbend poses work best if you have strengthened the muscles in your legs and buttocks by practising the standing poses regularly. Do the standing poses and/or several rounds of the *surya namaskar* (page 76) before doing backbends; this will warm you up and better enable you to arch your back. Focus on opening your upper chest rather than bending sharply from your lower back and follow up with a spinal twist or two.

SALABHASANA

LOCUST POSE

Salabhasana *promotes suppleness of the spine, strengthens the back muscles and opens up the chest. In some cases, this pose is recommended for slipped discs, but, if you do have such a condition, you must seek medical advice before practising any of the backbending poses.*

Equipment: blanket (optional).

Lie face down on the floor with your arms by your side and palms facing upwards. (You may want to place a blanket under your hips for comfort.) Keep your legs straight and together. Rest your forehead or chin on the floor.

Inhale and raise your arms, upper body and your legs, contracting the muscles in your buttocks. (In effect, you're balancing on your lower abdomen and pubis.) Firm your abdominal muscles.

Stretch you arms back towards your feet, parallel with the floor.

Stay in the raised position, breathing evenly, for about 10 breaths. (If you experience any back strain come out of the pose immediately.)

Exhale as you come down, and rest the head to one side.

Next, repeat the pose, but this time start with your legs bent and your feet parallel with the ceiling. Lift your upper body and your legs at the same time.

When you raise your upper body and legs, make sure you breathe evenly for the 10 breaths. Exhale as you come down.

If there is no back strain, repeat both variations, but don't increase the length of time you remain in the pose.

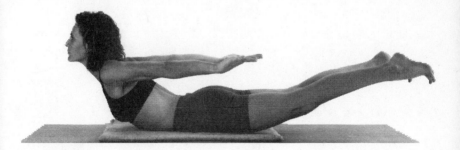

BHUJANGASANA

COBRA POSE

Practising bhujangasana regularly promotes back flexibility and strength. It also works the upper spine and opens the chest, increasing the ability to breathe deeply.

Lie face down with your legs straight and pressed together.

Place your palms on the floor under your shoulders and rest your forehead on the floor.

Press your pubic bone, legs and feet firmly into the floor. Draw back your abdomen.

Extend your chin forwards, then inhale slowly and lift your head, chest and abdomen, keeping your lower abdomen and pubis glued to the floor.

Breathe evenly in the elevated position.

Press down firmly on the inside of your hands to help you lift up.

With your shoulders moving down, take your head back and look up.

Lift your chest a little higher, but don't lift your hips or pubic bone off the floor.

Keep your buttocks firm.

Continue to breathe evenly for 10–15 breaths, and then exhale as you come down, stretching your chest forward as you descend.

Turn your head to the side, rest your arms alongside the body and breathe deeply.

Variation: If you want to challenge yourself more in the arch, start with your hands positioned beside your rib cage or even further back beside your hips. Press your tail-bone down and keep your buttocks and legs firm to avoid any pressure on your lower spine. This pose may be repeated.

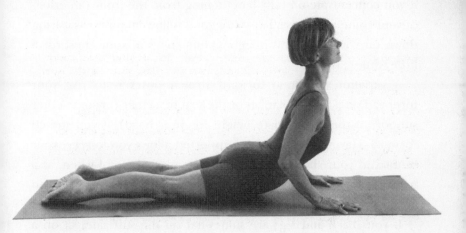

Forward stretches

Forward stretches are very good for soothing the nervous system and quietening the mind. It is more than likely that, as a beginner, you will have tight hamstrings, so go slowly, be patient and persevere.

Even though you seem to be stretching your back muscles (posterior spine) in these poses, you'll be working more effectively if you concentrate on fully lengthening from the front (anterior) of your spine and chest. Twists are good follow-on poses, as is lying down on your back and hugging your knees to your chest for a little while.

A variation on these forward stretch poses is to rest your forehead on a folded blanket or the seat of a chair (or some other support at the appropriate height for your head) as you stretch forward. Having the forehead supported allows you to relax your brain and your shoulders. This is particularly helpful when, as a novice, your hamstrings are resistant to stretching, or when you are feeling fatigued.

If your back and legs are somewhat on the stiff side, sit on a folded blanket for all the forward-stretching poses. Make sure the blanket is only under your buttocks, not the back of your thighs.

Keep a belt handy to use as an arm extender; you may need it to help you reach your foot without bowing your back.

FORWARD VIRASANA

HERO POSE STRETCHING FORWARD

This is an excellent pose to do at the beginning of your practice to stretch your back and loosen your hips. Forward virasana is a restful pose, and can be done anytime during your practice if you feel tired or light-headed.

Equipment: blanket or cushion (optional).

Start in the kneeling position you used for sitting *virasana* (page 62). Spread your knees apart and bring your big toes together so they touch. Your buttocks should be back towards or resting on your heels. If your buttocks don't quite reach your heels, place a folded blanket or cushion between your heels and your buttocks.

Bend your body forwards and stretch your arms out in front of you. Press your hands down with your fingers spread.

Extend your arms, waist and chest forwards, but don't hunch your shoulders.

Rest your forehead on the floor or on a folded blanket. Stay in this pose for 1–3 minutes, breathing evenly and relaxing your shoulders.

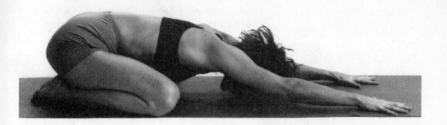

JANU SIRSASANA

HEAD-TO-KNEE POSE

This forward stretch tones the liver, spleen and kidneys, as well as stretching the back leg muscles. Although the Sanscrit translation of janu sirasana is 'head to knee', that is not a good goal for beginners!

Equipment: belt.

Sit on the floor with your legs stretched straight in front of you. Keep the left leg straight and bend the right leg in, so your knee is at a right angle to your right hip. The heel of your right foot should be near the top of the left groin, with the sole of your foot facing up. Check that you're not sitting on your right foot.

Place your hands beside your hips and adjust your hips so that they are square and level. Turn your trunk towards the left, so your breastbone is in line with the centre of your left leg.

Loop the belt over the ball of your left foot, one hand holding each side of the belt. Gradually, over a few cycles of deep breathing, hold the belt a little closer to the foot or, if you can, hold your foot.

Make sure that you keep your spine straight, not bowing. Lift your chest, and tuck your chin in slightly to extend the back of your neck.

While you're in this pose, concentrate on turning your navel to the left and keeping your right buttock on the floor.

Only hold your foot if you are able to hold both sides of it without bowing your back or bending your left leg.

Keep moving your shoulders down and keep the muscles in your back soft.

Hold the extension for about 1 minute, then reverse the position of the legs and repeat all the adjustments on the right side.

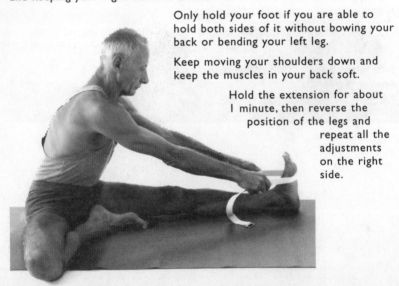

PASCHIMOTTANASANA
THE GREAT WESTERN STRETCH

The word paschima *means 'the west' and implies the back of the body (the front of the body is the east). In paschimottanasana, the whole back of the body is given an intense stretch. This pose is good for extending the spine and the backs of the legs. Additionally, it tones the abdominal organs and the kidneys.*

Equipment: blanket (optional); belt.

Sit on the floor or, if you are a little stiff, on a folded blanket.

Stretch your legs out straight in front of you and keep your feet and legs together.

Place the belt over the balls of your feet, holding it with both hands. Pull back a little on the belt and sit up straight.

Begin to work your hands up the belt a little further and extend your trunk outwards, not down. Only consider moving your hands closer to your feet if your spine is not bowing.

Lift the front of your chest up, and move your shoulders and the back of your chest down towards your buttocks. Keep your legs straight and the inside of your legs and knees rotating inwards.

Tuck your chin in slightly to extend the back of your neck.

If you are supple, you may be able to hold the sides of your feet, or even catch hold of your wrist behind the soles of your feet.

Stay in the pose for 1–3 minutes, breathing evenly.

Inhale and come up slowly.

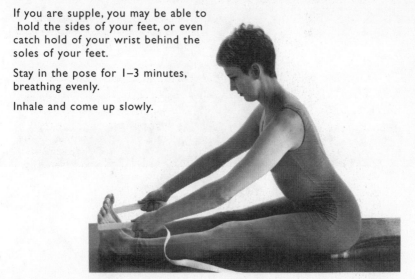

UPAVISTHA KONASANA

SPLITS

Upavistha konasana *gives a tremendous stretch to the inside of the legs, particularly the groins and knees. It is a soothing pose to do during menstruation, especially if the head is supported on a chair or on folded blankets. And it's just what the midwife ordered, along with* baddha konasana *(page 64), to help pregnant women, although women in their second or third trimester of pregnancy should avoid doing supine* upavistha konasana *(Variation 2).*

Equipment: blanket or chair.

Sit on the floor with your buttocks lifted onto a folded blanket.

Spread your legs wide enough apart so that you are challenged, but not so wide that your hamstrings and groins feel pain.

Place your hands behind your buttocks and press your fingertips down to help lift your trunk upwards.

Keep your knees and thigh muscles pulled up, and press the backs of your knees towards the floor. Your feet should be perpendicular, resting on the centre of your heels, with your toes pointed up towards the ceiling.

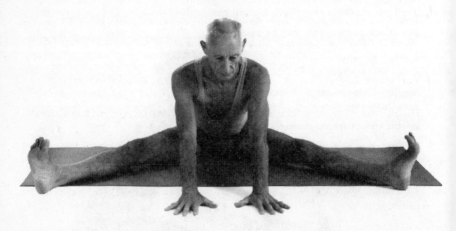

If your hamstrings and the muscles in your back will allow, place your hands in front of your body and stretch forwards. If your back begins to bow, return to a more upright position with your hands behind your buttocks.

Hold the pose for about 1–2 minutes, then bend your knees and bring your legs together.

Variation 1: To do a lateral stretch and twist in the pose, remain in the splits position. Press your hands to the floor on either side of your right leg to help you lift and turn your trunk towards your right leg.

Loop a belt over your right foot, hold both ends of the belt in your left hand and, with your right hand still on the outside of your right leg, press down to help keep your right chest lifted. Continue turning towards the right. Keep your left buttock and left leg flush to the floor as you rotate to the right. Keep stretching and turning towards the right and extending your spine upwards.

If it is easy for you to catch hold of the outside of your right foot with your left hand, do so, but keep your shoulders down.

Hold the pose for 1 minute, breathing evenly.

Turn back to the centre and repeat the adjustments on the left side.

To come out of the pose, bend your knees and bring your legs together.

Variation 2: If your back is tight or sore, you may benefit from doing this pose lying down.

Lie on your back near to a wall. Bend your legs and wiggle your buttocks as close as you can to the wall.

Straighten your legs and move them wide apart into the splits. Adjust your feet so they are equidistant from the floor. Work on straightening your legs by pulling up your kneecaps.

Your arms can be loose by the side of your body or loosely folded over your head.

Hold the pose for 3–5 minutes, breathing evenly.

Twists

Twists are effective counterposes for most other poses. They undo the little kinks we may inadvertently put in our back while exercising.

Twisting the spine is rarely a natural movement in the course of a normal day. The spine can therefore become misaligned, and the ribs and spine can become stiff and brittle.

To improve flexibility in the spine, ribs and back muscles, twists should be included in your yoga practice as often as possible.

It is quite tempting to hold your breath while practising twists, because you are turning the diaphragm as well as your spine. Therefore, as you go in to the twist, breathe in, extend your spine, then exhale and turn, breathe in, extend, exhale and turn, over several cycles of breathing. Your breathing will enhance the twisting movement and you will be more conscious of the need to breathe.

If you are pregnant, do only gentle twists that do not put pressure on your abdomen. Similarly, if you are menstruating, avoid any poses that put pressure on your lower abdomen. Finally, do not practice twists if you have displaced discs.

CHAIR TWIST

A twist a day could keep your chiropractor at bay. The chair twist is one of the most valuable exercises for your back. You may have intuitively discovered this pose already. Many office workers tend to do it when they realise that they've been sitting for some time without taking a break. The chair twist releases tension in the back muscles and helps to realign the spine after long periods of studying or working at a computer.

Equipment: straight-backed chair.

Sit sideways on a straight-backed chair, with your right hip towards the back of the chair.

Sit right back to the edge of the chair, with both feet flat on the floor. Ensure your knees and feet are slightly apart.

Place both hands on the back of the chair, one each side. Keep your hips and knees in a straight line.

Pull with your left hand to help you turn the left side of your body around towards the back of the chair. Use your right hand to help you turn the right side of your body away from the back of the chair.

Let your neck rotate to look back over your right shoulder, but don't force your neck, if it feels stiff.

Check to see your knees and hips are still in a straight line. (Your left hip will want to come forward.)

With several longer exhalations, use the out-breaths to help you turn your trunk even further around to the right. Keep your breastbone lifting and your spine stretching up, but your shoulders moving down.

Hold the position for about 10–15 breaths, then release.

Repeat all the above adjustments on the other side, seated with your left hip towards the back of the chair and turning to your left side.

If the chair twist feel like a good release for your back, you can do it twice.

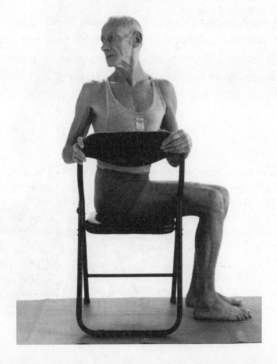

SUKHASANA TWIST

EASY CROSSED-LEGGED TWIST

This is the simplest of twists and can be a good way to start a practice, after supta baddha kosana or virisana, as it eliminates stiffness in the back muscles.

Equipment: blanket.

Sit on a folded blanket with your legs loosely crossed. Press your hands down next to your hips and lift your spine upwards. Place your left hand on your right knee and your right hand on the floor behind your buttocks.

Pull on your right knee to help you turn your trunk towards the right. Keep your chest lifted, your shoulders down and your left buttock pressed to the floor. Use your breath to help you turn: inhale and stretch up, exhale and turn. Do this several times.

Release your hands and turn back to the centre.

Reverse the way you crossed your legs and repeat the twist, this time placing your right hand on your left knee, your left hand behind you, and turning to the left side.

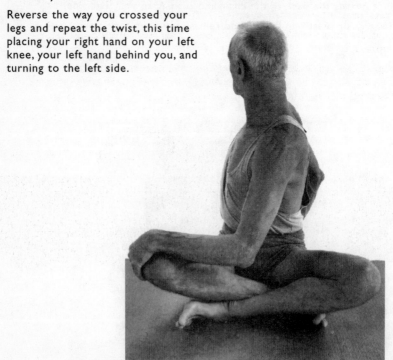

ARDHA JATHARA PARIVARTANASANA

BELLY TWISTER

This pose is very good for alleviating stiffness in the back and back-ache. It also gives a gentle massage to the abdominal organs (you will need blankets or cushions set up on either side of your hips if you are tight in the shoulders or hips.)

Equipment: 2 blankets or 2 cushions (optional).

Lie down on your back and stretch your arms out sideways so they are in line with your shoulders, palms up.

Bend your knees into your chest. Exhale and take your knees down to floor on the right side, pointing towards the right armpit.

If your knees don't quite touch the floor, let your bent legs rest on a folded blanket or cushion to the right side.

Keep extending your left arm and revolving your abdomen to the left. Press your left shoulder down if it is lifting off the floor.

Hold the pose for 15–20 breaths, then bring your knees back to the centre again.

Repeat the pose, this time taking your knees down to the left side. Hold the pose for 15–20 breaths, then bring your knees back to the centre. Repeat the pose once more on each side.

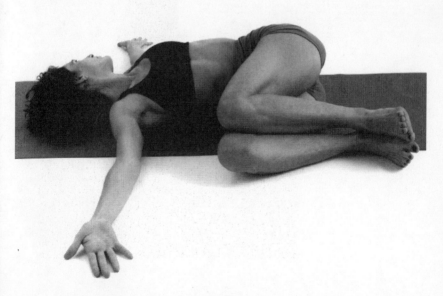

Restorative poses

The restorative poses in yoga help to refresh you when you are tired, suffering from jet lag or recovering from illness. Even if you practised only *supta baddha konasana*, *viparita karani* and *savasana* for 10 minutes each, without doing any other poses, you would recharge your energy quite considerably. These poses are 'cost-effective' in terms of putting in minimum effort for maximum renewal of energy.

SUPTA BADDHA KONASANA
BOUND-ANGLE POSE

Since this pose is practised lying down, it is very restful and therapeutic. It helps you to centre, and is beneficial during pregnancy and for cramps arising from menstruation. It also tones the kidneys. If your groins are tight, baddha konasana will gradually loosen them.

Equipment: 2 blankets or a bolster and a blanket; eye bag (optional).

Lie back on a bolster or a blanket folded lengthwise to support your back and head. Place another blanket under your head and neck for comfort.

Bend your knees out sideways and bring the soles of your feet together, bringing your heels as close to the pubis as possible.

Let your back settle and your chest open.

Stretch your knees towards the floor.

Take your arms out to the side and rest them beside your trunk, palms up. If you do not experience shoulder tension, you can rest your arms loosely overhead.

As a beginner, stay in position for 1–5 minutes, breathing evenly, with your eyes closed. You may wish to cover your eyes with an eye bag. With more experience, you can stay in position for up to 10 minutes.

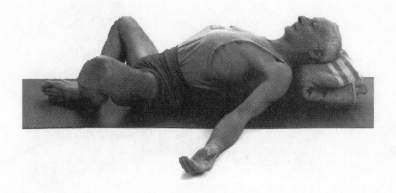

VIPARITA KARANI

LEGS-UP-THE-WALL POSE

This simple pose is one that people often do instinctively to alleviate tiredness in the legs or lower backache. It helps bring extra circulation to the upper body because you are in an inverted position and it nourishes the nervous system.

Equipment: blanket (optional); eye bag or cloth.

Lie on your back, near to a wall, with your legs bent. Wiggle in as close as you can, until your buttocks are flush to the wall. Stretch your legs straight up and let the wall support them.

If you find that your lower back is rounding or that your buttocks are lifting off the floor, move your buttocks slightly further away from the wall. You may want to support your head and neck on a folded blanket for greater comfort.

Rest your arms loosely overhead or alongside your body, palms upward, if your shoulders are tight.

Stay in this pose for 5–20 minutes, breathing evenly, with your eyes covered by a soft cloth or eye bag.

When you're ready to release the pose, bend your legs in, roll to one side, and take your time to come up.

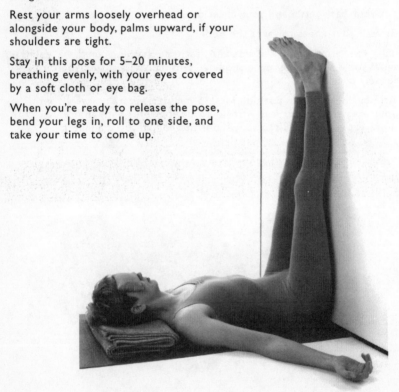

Variation: *Viparita karani* with legs on a chair (pictured below) is a good pose to do when you don't have the space to put your legs up a wall. It is also an excellent restorative pose in its own right.

Lie down and lift your lower legs onto the seat of the chair. Move your buttocks in close to the chair and rest your arms by your side. Support the back of your head and neck with a folded blanket. Cover your eyes with an eye bag or soft cloth. Stay in the pose for 5–15 minutes. You will find your breathing becomes very gentle and quiet.

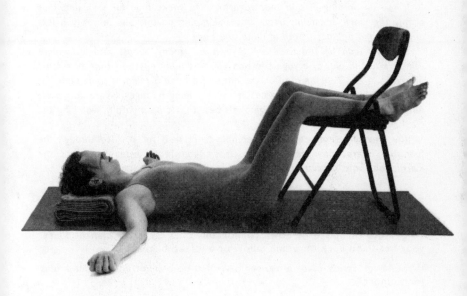

SAVASANA

CORPSE POSE

Sava (pronounced 'shava') is the Sanskrit for corpse. The image of a corpse is used to make us to think of the ultimate state of letting go, of the total stillness that comes with death, and also of surrendering all thoughts of the past, even of the yoga practice you have been doing. The intention is to feel complete and present in the moment.

I can't really say enough good things about the yoga relaxation. All the benefits you would expect from deep relaxation are available in savasana: release of muscular tension, reduction of fatigue, a boost for the immune system, a levelling out of blood pressure (whether it is too high or too low), and a lowering of the heart rate.

If you do nothing else in your yoga practice, make time for savasana. It is simply the single most important pose. Skimping on this one leaves you less energetic and balanced, both in mind and body.

Savasana can be practised on its own, but many people find it is more effective at the end of a yoga practice. The optimum length of time to remain in savasana can be estimated on the basis of around 5 minutes (minimum) for every 30 minutes of yoga practice. Of course, doing a longer savasana is quite alright any time. As you can imagine, it's best to not be mentally 'watching the clock'.

You may find that you are better able to relax if you are led through the following instructions step by step. If so, you many want to record the instructions on a cassette tape.

Equipment: 1–2 blankets; pillow (optional); bolster (optional); cloth or eye bag (optional).

To get into this pose, lie down comfortably on a carpet or blanket. Place your head and neck on a thin pillow or a folded blanket.

If your back aches, place a bolster or rolled-up blanket under your knees for support.

Depending on the weather, you may want an extra blanket to cover your body, because you will find that your body temperature drops quite significantly during the relaxation.

Lift your head for just a moment and look at the front of your body — your chin, breastbone and pubic bone should be in one straight line. If they are not, adjust your position. Lower your head onto the blanket again, resting your head on the very centre of the back of your skull.

Close your eyes now and, if you wish, cover them with a soft cloth or an eye bag. Having a light weight on the eyes when they are closed helps them to relax quickly and blocks out any light.

Adjust your arms so they are equidistant from your body, about 15 cm away from the side ribs. Rotate your arms outwards from the shoulders until your palms are facing the ceiling. Press your arms gently into the floor to help you lift up the back chest a little and lower it again so that the right and left sides of your back rest evenly on the floor and your shoulder blades are flat. Relax your arms and hands. Soften the skin on your palms and relax your fingers so they are loose.

Let your legs fall naturally to the sides, with your feet a comfortable distance apart and rolling out gently. Soften the skin on the soles of your feet.

Now, mentally scan the body to locate and release any areas of tension. The most common trouble spots are the buttocks and lower back, the abdomen and diaphragm, and the neck and shoulders. You may notice that, even though you've relaxed your face, it still feels 'pinched', or your forehead may seem furrowed. Relax them, as well as the roof and the floor of your mouth, your lips and your jaw.

Relax your facial muscles. Soften the skin on your forehead and temples, and imagine your brain relaxing back from your forehead and resting towards the back of your skull.

Relax all the tiny muscles around your eyes and relax your eyes so that they sink back in their sockets.

Soften your tongue and let it relax to the back lower palate, away from your teeth.

Now that your eyes are relaxed, you can 'look' down and inwards to observe the movement of your breath in your chest and abdomen.

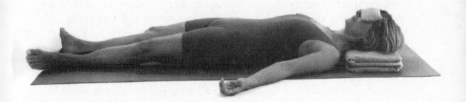

Take several conscious breaths, inhaling deeply and exhaling just as deeply. Be aware of the rising of your chest and abdomen with each inhalation, and the falling of your chest and abdomen with each exhalation. Then let your breath find its natural, steady rhythm.

Let your breath become more and more gentle and rhythmical. Breathe quietly. Maintain a faint awareness of your body and your breath, so that you don't drift off or fall asleep.

As your mind quietens, imagine it sinking with the exhalation phase of your breath in the centre of your chest. Repeat over several successive exhalations.

To keep your mind from drifting off, stay focused on your breath, until you notice it becoming quite subtle and smooth.

Let your thoughts come to a complete standstill.

Your body and senses are at rest. Your mind is at rest. There is a pervasive feeling of balance and harmony, and your breath has subsided to its minimum, like the ebb tide.

Remain motionless, enjoying your peace of mind, for about 10 minutes or longer, and then, when you want to come out, bend your left knee, stretch your right arm out to the side and roll onto your right side. Just let your eye covering fall off. Let your eyes open gradually and become accustomed to the light.

Remain motionless a moment longer. Feel your whole body and your breath, and the peaceful state of your mind. Move slowly into a sitting position. Take a further moment, seated comfortably, to check that you are fully in your body; aware of your physical sensations and your breath. Enjoy how the relaxation has made you feel.

Twelve-Week Program

In this section, I have put together a series of lessons that will take your through a 12-week period of yoga practice. They include all the poses described here in this book.

On alternate days of the first week, do lessons 1 and 2. In the second week, do lessons 2 and 3; in the third week, lessons 3 and 4; and so on up to week 12. In week 12, on alternate days, do lesson 12 and those poses you have found to be most challenging. By the end of week 12 you will have completed all the lessons and all the poses. This repetition ensures you will consolidate a small number of poses in a short time. Only when you have mastered the basics do you move forward to build on what you have learned. Your progress will obviously be proportionate to how often and how long you practice, as well as to the level of fitness you have to begin with.

LESSON 1

- *supta baddha konasana*
- forward *virasana*
- right-angle stretch
- *tadasana*
- *urdhva hastasana*
- *trikonasana*
- *virabhadrasana II*
- *uttanasana*
- *virasana*
- *sukhasana* twist
- *savasana*

(**Note:** When doing standing poses as a beginner, it is good practice to do them twice.)

LESSON 2

- *supta baddha konasana*
- forward *virasana*
- right-angle stretch
- chest-opener
- *tadasana*
- *trikonasana*
- *virabhadrasana II*
- *parsvakonasana*
- *uttanasana*
- *gommukhasana*
- chair twist
- *savasana*

(**Note:** If you experience any back pain in *uttanasana*, replace it with the right-angle stretch.)

LESSON 3

- *supta baddha konasana*
- *sukhasana* twist
- chest-opener
- *adho mukha svanasana*
- *uttanasana*
- *tadasana*
- *trikonasana* × 2
- *virabhadrasana II* × 2
- *parsvakonasana* × 2
- *parsvottanasana* × 2
- *janu sirsasana*
- *sukhasana*
- *viparita karani*
- *savasana*

(**Note:** Begin to develop more arm strength in the standing poses by keeping your arms extended, even when you do the second side.)

LESSON 4

- *virasana*
- forward *virasana*
- chest-opener
- *adho mukha svanasana*
- *uttanasana*
- *tadasana*
- *urdhva hastasana*
- *trikonasana*
- *parsvakonasana*
- *uttanasana*
- *parsvakonasana*
- *prasarita padottanasana*
- *uttanasana*
- *supta baddha konasana*
- *baddha konasana*, seated
- *janu sirsasana*
- *savasana*

(**Note:** Do the standing poses with the heel of the back foot pressing against a wall or skirting board, to give you a greater sensation of stretching the muscles of the back leg.)

LESSON 5

- *viparita karani*
- open your legs into *upavistha konasana*, with your legs still on the wall from *viparita karani*
- right-angle stretch
- *adho mukha svanasana*
- *uttanasana*
- *adho mukha svanasana*
- *uttanasana*
- *adho mukha svanasana*
- lunge × 2
- *adho mukha svanasana*
- *uttanasana*
- *virasana*
- forward *virasana*
- *gommukhasana*
- *paripurna navasana* × 2
- *sukhasana* twist
- *savasana*

(**Note:** Do *adho mukha svanasana* and the lunges with your heels pressing against the wall to stretch your legs more.)

LESSON 6

- *supta baddha konasana*
- *baddha konasana,* seated
- *adho mukha svanasana* x 2
- lunge x 2
- *uttanasana*
- *tadasana* x 2
- *urdhva hastasana* x 2
- *trikonasana* x 2
- *virabhadrasana II* x 2
- *parsvakonasana* x 2
- *prasarita padottanasana* x 2
- *virasana*
- *salabhasana*
- *bhujangasana*
- chair twist
- chair *viparita karani*
- *savasana*

(**Note:** Do *trikonasana* and *virabhadrasana II* with the back of your body against a wall to check your alignment is correct.)

LESSON 7

- *virasana*
- forward *virasana*
- *adho mukha svanasana*
- lunge
- *uttanasana*
- *urdhva hastasana*
- *tadasana*
- *urdhva hastasana*
- *uttanasana*
- *urdhva hastasana*
- *tadasana*
- *surya namaskar* x 5
- *virasana*
- *bhujangasana*
- *salabhasana*
- *bhujangasana*
- forward *virasana*
- *sukhasana* twist
- *paschimottanasana*
- *savasana*

(**Note:** With *surya namaskar*, keep checking that you are breathing in rhythm with your movement and that your alignment is correct, even though you're only holding each pose for one inhalation or exhalation.)

LESSON 8

- *supta baddha konasana*
- *baddha konasana,* seated
- *gommukhasana*
- *supta padangusthasana* cycle
- chest-opener
- *tadasana*
- *trikonasana*
- *virabhadrasana II*
- *parsvakonasana*
- *parsvottanasana,* with variation (hands in 'prayer' position)
- *prasarita padottanasana,* with variation (hands interlocked behind you)
- *uttanasana*
- chair twist
- *janu sirasana*
- *viparita karani*
- *savasana*

(**Note:** Hold the *supta padangusthasana* variations for 15 long breaths each and keep the legs very straight to enhance the stretch.)

LESSON 9

- forward *virasana*
- *sukhasana*
- *adho mukha svanasana*
- *uttanasana*
- lunge x 2
- *surya namaskar* x 10
- *virasana*
- *paripurna navasana* x 2
- *janu sirsansana*
- *upavistha konasana* forward stretch
- *upavistha konasana* twist
- *paschimottanasana*
- *ardha jatara parivartanasana*
- *viparita karani*
- *savasana*

(**Note:** Build up to longer timings in *adho mukha svanasana*, *uttanasana* and the lunge, to improve stamina and flexibility. Use your breath as a guide, and if your breathing becomes rough, you may need to rest until your breath becomes smooth again.)

LESSON 10

- *virasana*
- forward *virasana*
- *adho mukha svanasana*
- *uttanasana*
- *adho mukha svanasana*
- *uttanasana*
- *tadasana*
- *urdhava hastasana* to *uttanasana* x 10
- right-angle stretch
- *paripurna navasana*
- *bhujangasana* x 2
- *salabasana* x 2
- *supta padangusthasana* cycle
- *ardha jatara parivartanasana*
- chair *viparita karani*
- *savasana*

(**Note:** In the backbends, make sure you are stretching the breastbone up, tucking in the shoulder blades and keeping your abdominal muscles and buttocks firm.)

LESSON 11

- *supta baddha konasana*
- *baddha konasana*, seated
- *gommukhasana*
- chest-opener
- *adho mukha svanasana*
- *uttanasana*
- *tadasana*
- *urdhva hastasana*
- *trikonasana*
- *virabhadrasana II*
- *parsvakonasana*
- *parsvottanasana* (do the 'prayer' position variation the second time)
- *prasarita padottanasana* (do the arm stretch variation the second time)
- *uttanasana*
- *paripurna navasana*
- *virasana*
- chair twist
- *savasana*

(**Note:** In this practice, run through all standing poses once, holding for 20–30 seconds each, then repeat them.)

LESSON 12

(RESTORATIVE SEQUENCE)

- *supta baddha konasana*
- forward *virasana*
- *baddha konasana*, forward stretch
- *gommukhasana*
- *adho mukha svanasana* (with the crown of your head resting on cushions, blankets or a block)
- *uttanasana* (with your head and arms resting on the seat of a chair, buttocks on the wall and feet 20cm from the wall)
- *supta padangusthasana* cycle
- *janu sirsasana* (head supported on a bolster, blankets or the seat of a chair)
- *paschimottanasana* (head supported on a bolster, blankets or the seat of a chair)
- *sukhasana* twist
- *upavistha konasana* legs on the wall
- chair *viparita karani*
- *savasana*

(**Note:** Especially when doing a restorative sequence, it is beneficial to keep your eyes covered in the lying-down poses.)

6 THE YOGA OF STRESS REDUCTION

Not everyone wants to have less stress in their lives. Some people apparently thrive on stress!

A dear friend of mine used to say that he loved yoga because it gave him the energy to accomplish more than he ever had before. And he was already doing more than two or three people put together! Some people worry about burning out; he was more concerned about 'rusting' out. Twelve yoga years later, I'm pleased to say, he has dramatically simplified his life; he still accomplishes more than most, but in a more relaxed way.

Stress is a part of life, and there are many advantages to living in the accelerated, intense pace of the late 20th century. It is how we've created our miraculous, civilised world. Our cities grow at an unbelievable rate. High-rises mushroom up from vacant lots in what seems like a couple of months. Our competitive economic system means we can choose from myriad products, and we have a mindset that constantly strives for the state-of-the-art. Opportunities in every sphere are countless, if only you have enough imagination and persistence.

So why do we hear of so many people who want to 'jump ship'? Like the American transcendentalist H.D. Thoreau, who secluded himself at Walden Pond, these folk want to move to the country. They want to decrease their work hours, stop work altogether or rediscover the simple things in life, a view that seems almost old fashioned now. Thoreau exhorted his 19th-century contemporaries to 'Simplify, simplify … Our life is frittered away by detail'. Is this simpler lifestyle actually our birthright, and not really old-fashioned at all? I believe that this is part of the reason why people are turning to the ancient traditions like yoga — to help them find some peace of mind and a measure of wisdom.

Not all the progress we are making supports our everyday lives; our souls' needs are not being met. Do you ever ask yourself, 'Why am I doing this?', or 'Why do I do it this way?', or even 'Why bother?'. Have you noticed that when you have a weekend off or a holiday that these questions often come up, but just as often don't get resolved? After the break, it's back to business as usual.

Over the years, I have developed skilful ways of eliminating the stresses that arise in my own daily life. I believe they will help you, too. They are:

1 slow down
2 plan your time
3 train your attention
4 find inspiring books and friends
5 'don't do something, sit there'
6 see the bigger picture

Reducing stress doesn't happen all at once. I'm still on a learning curve as I interweave these insights into my own yoga practice. At the same time, my yoga practice tends to feed back its own wisdom. If these principles strike a chord with you, use them to support yourself in your yoga and your life. Hopefully you will then find you have more energy and more 'mental space' which can be directed towards the common good.

Slow down

If there is just one change you can make in your thoughts and actions to turn your life around, I believe it would be to *slow down*.

Regular relaxation is a crucial part of learning to slow down. Every time you practice yoga relaxation, you are learning to listen to your own rhythm.

Our hurried, harried pace is so much a part of our expression, it's like the very air we breathe. We're not genetically coded to rush constantly, but 'the urgency addiction' seems to have become second nature to us.

'Hurry up!' is an injunction that many of us have embodied from a very early age. Even when there are no external demands being made on us, there is still a feeling of internal pressure to make haste. Have you noticed how you'll jump into your car at the beginning of a holiday exodus and speed off, and go right on speeding, even when you have no timetable to adhere to? It's a sad state of affairs that on a two-week break, we need a week of it to slow down!

In 10-day *vipassana* meditation retreats, one technique used to slow people down is walking meditation, which is done in periodic one-hour sessions throughout the day. An outsider watching a meditator doing this practice may find the slow walking has an eerie, zombie-like quality. This is simply because the meditator is paying infinitesimal attention to the details of something we usually do completely mechanically. The mind is humbled when you stop to observe the minute adjustments the body makes every time you take a step. When the mind is focused like this, as it is in your yoga practice, mind chatter slows down dramatically, or even stops. It is ultimately very calming.

It is up to you whether you want to relax and slow down. But understand that it really is okay to slow down. Sometimes the thought of slowing down is so revolutionary, so unfamiliar, even scary, that you have to talk yourself into it. Reassure yourself that it's okay to stop, take your time and breathe, and even to sit down and think about what *you* want or need. The underlying message is: *you matter.*

Plan your time

I was never much of a planner until I became involved with some events that required good organisation. They went so much more smoothly because of my planning that I had the time and energy to really enjoy them. (One of these events involved my wedding plans!) At worst, good planning can prevent inelegant outcomes. At best, it can support your entire wellbeing and perhaps save you more time in the long run.

Start your day earlier, as I recommended when discussing the best time to do your yoga practice. This means your quiet time is guaranteed. People tell me that they have more energy as a result of getting up early, because they're doing something purely ('selfishly'!) for themselves.

Create a generous, regular period of free time for your yoga practice, meditation, inspirational reading, journal writing, reflection or even doing nothing. There's an art to doing absolutely nothing, as you learn from being in yoga relaxation. Don't let anything rob you of this invaluable part of the day.

If you know that you won't be able to take a holiday for quite some time, consider taking short breaks more frequently. My husband Daniel and I have an agreement to go away for the weekend once a month. Your trip need not be expensive: visit your friends in the country, or swap houses with them on the weekend, or go camping.

If you can't get away, even for a weekend, create everyday breathing space by having a 'holi-hour' — a once-a-day break to do whatever you like that is a non work or non family-oriented activity. Go for a walk on the beach or in the park.

Take the time to treat yourself to a healthy breakfast. Stop to enjoy all your meals, without eating on the run. There will always be more to be done!

Eat with gratitude. It's a great digestive.

Be guided in what you choose to eat by what is good for your body, not just good to taste. This change occurs naturally the more you connect with your body through yoga practice.

Organise yourself well enough to allow plenty of time to get to every appointment, even if it means you arrive a little early, so you can enjoy the travel.

Treat yourself with respect. Constantly flogging yourself to do more and more is a subtle form of self-abuse.

Respect those close to you, too. Don't put pressure on the people you live and work with to dance to your tempo.

Look for ways to make your life simpler. Periodically, assess what you do in your routine and stop doing those things that are unnecessary, unfulfilling or even disempowering. I call this practice 'green-bagging' — the process of cleaning out your overcrowded closet and garage. It affords you the same kind mental space.

On the other hand, hold fast to those activities that make your heart sing.

You nourish your body by eating good-quality food and exercising regularly. Nourish your mind, too, through all your senses. Choose good-quality input in what you read, watch and listen to. We are what we think. What goes in to you through your senses becomes part of who you are.

Reduce the amount of time you spend relating to electronic equipment: computers, faxes, mobile phones, televisions and radios. At our annual summer yoga retreat, besides the country setting, wholesome food and doing lots of yoga, another soothing aspect is that we are 'unplugged'. There is nothing that beeps and buzzes, talks at us or intrudes on our quietude.

Use your new-found ambling pace to pay more attention to detail; to notice everyday miracles and the changing fragrances of the seasons.

Train your attention

Many longtime practitioners would describe their yoga as 'awareness training' — practising to be in the here and now. Even though this is done through the vehicle of the body, it is very much a harnessing of the mind. The following suggestions reinforce what you are learning through practising yoga.

* Stop trying to do more than one thing at a time. In your yoga practice, you develop the ability to concentrate and this skill helps create composure. Cultivate a sense of self-assurance and wellbeing by focusing your attention on the moment.

* Break the 'juggling act' habit. Why create so much stress in your life by trying to keep all those balls in the air, especially when many of them may end up on the floor? Focus on the one thing on your plate, complete as much as you can and then move on to the next thing.

* Bring the patience and attentiveness that you develop in your yoga practice into your personal relationships. When you're with someone, give them all your attention.

* When you're driving a car, give your full attention to the road. This a very

mundane meditation, but an effective one. It is alarming how often you get caught in a reverie and drive from point A to point B without ever being aware of the traffic or the environment on the way.

* Make work work for you. Nowadays, with many of us working from our homes, it's harder to draw the line between work and the rest of our lives. So we end up feeling that we're never completely at work or at home.

   This problem comes up in your yoga, too. Train yourself to do only your practice when you're practising, instead of finding, all of a sudden, that you're making a cup of tea or hanging out a load of washing. Deal with outside distractions by setting strict time and space boundaries and sticking to them.

* When you're at work give it your full attention, and when you're with your family give them your full attention. Avoid bringing office projects or politics home, either in your head or in your briefcase.

* If your attention ever gets stuck in a pattern of obsessive thinking, throw yourself into something that requires all of your concentration, such as doing very detailed work or a strong yoga practice.

   Everything you take on should be worthy of your attention. If you are doing something and finding that you're only partially attentive, ask yourself: Is this task really worth doing?

Find inspiring books and friends

Reading the newspapers and listening to the television news, we sometimes end up feeling resigned or depressed. Generally speaking, the media doesn't portray the world and its inhabitants in a favourable light. An antidote to this, and an altogether uplifting tonic, is daily reading from the 'wisdom literature' — the philosophic, proverbial and religious literature that teaches the art of living — especially if you read it in the early morning to give you an inspiring start to the day, or before bed, to inspire your dreams.

Spend plenty of time with friends and mentors, those kindred spirits whose company makes you feel better. Get together often with close friends. Fun and laughter can be profoundly healing.

Make each encounter you have more personal and respectful, whether it's with the newsagent, the waiter or your relationship partner.

When Indians greet each other, they join their hands over their hearts in a prayerful gesture and say '*Namaste*'. It means 'The divine spark in me salutes the divinity in you'. If we mentally make this small but significant gesture with each person we come in contact with, it helps us to spread goodwill and to be less impersonal. We feel better about ourselves and the other person.

'Don't just do something, sit there'

Learn to make meditation part of your life and fit it in whenever you can. The perfect time to sit in meditation is after having done a yoga practice, when the body and mind are at their quietest. Or mediate first thing in the morning, as early as possible, when you are unlikely to be disturbed. It also works well to meditate late in the evening, as it helps to foster a peaceful sleep.

I've set aside a special place that I use for my quiet time. Being in this space helps me feel tranquil straight away.

The simplest way to meditate is to sit comfortably with your spine erect, either in a straight-back chair or cross-legged on the floor with your back against a wall. Close your eyes and focus on your breathing. This basic technique, called *zazen*, meaning 'just sitting', has been practised by Buddhist monks for centuries.

Don't let yourself get caught up in following a stream of thoughts or drifting off, just focus on your breath. You will be distracted from time to time, especially if you're new to meditation. Don't let this upset you: just go back to focusing on your breath. When your mind goes off at a tangent again, gently come back to the breath.

Most of all, use this time to cultivate patience and peace.

The bigger picture

Ultimately, I believe, one's personal practices carry over into the public sphere. The healthy choices you make for yourself, such as doing a regular yoga practice, contribute to the wellbeing of others every bit as much as to yourself.

One characteristic of mature yoga practice is that the energy you generate for yourself and your own healing can be directed outwards towards humanity and the planet.

When you quieten your constant mind chatter, you are able to think and see far more clearly. This enables you to evaluate situations objectively and, because your mind is disciplined, you know what needs to be done (or not done) to make your unique contribution to life.

In summary, there are many things to attend to when you're learning yoga, the most important of which are your attitude and your awareness. Developing these is a process that is simple, but not necessarily easy. It is, after all, life training, as you have seen. You are building up a muscle for taking care of yourself on all levels — body, mind and spirit. In the beginning, especially, you have to work at it, but the rewards are great. Persevere.

ABOUT THE YOGA MODELS

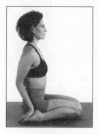

SOO BALBI, 34

Soo is a devoted mother, wife, award-winning advertising art director, painter, writer and skating enthusiast. Yoga provides the foundation that makes the rest of her life work. She has been studying Iyengar yoga for 9 years, practices a couple of hours a day and teaches at the Sydney Yoga Centre. Through yoga, Soo has overcome a serious back problem which medical specialists said would leave her disabled.

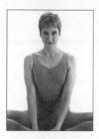

MARDI KENDALL, 42

Mardi hails from the American Midwest, and lived in California, Scotland and Paris before moving to Australia in 1989. Her diverse careers of cellist, model and Shiatsu practitioner find their present balance in teaching yoga and co-directing the Sydney Yoga Centres. Her teaching is well known for its compelling combination of humour, compassion and embracing the transformative possibilities of yoga.

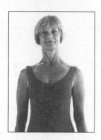

EVE GRZYBOWSKI, 52

Eve, the author of this book, has been a yoga practitioner since 1971 and has studied with Martyn Jackson and B.K.S. Iyengar. A yoga teacher since 1980, she teaches yoga students and trains yoga teachers at the Sydney Yoga Centre, which she founded in 1985.

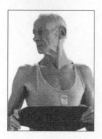

COLLYN RIVERS, 67

Collyn was born in North Africa and came of age in England. He has worked as an engineer, writer and publisher. Collyn started yoga in his late 50s, proving that transformation can occur at any age. Having practised now for over 15 years, he boasts the heart rate of a marathon runner. Severe inherited back problems brought him to yoga and eventually the co-directorship of the Sydney Yoga Centre, where he never ceases to amaze and inspire his students.

BIBLIOGRAPHY

Bhagavad Gita, translated by Eknath Easwaran, Nilgiri Press, 1985.

J.C. Chatterji, *The Wisdom of the Vedas*, Quest Books, 1992.

Stephen R. Covey, *The Seven Habits of Highly Effective People*, Simon & Schuster, New York, 1990.

— —, *First Things First*, Simon & Schuster, New York, 1994.

T.K.V. Desikachar, *The Heart of Yoga*, Inner Traditions International, Vermont, 1995.

— —, *The Yoga of T. Krishnamacharya*, Krishnamacharya Yoga Mandiram, Madras, 1982.

— —, *Patanjali's Yoga-Sutras*, Affiliated East-West Press, New Delhi, 1987.

Donna Farhi, *The Breathing Book*, Henry Holt Publishers, New York, 1996.

B.K.S. Iyengar, *Light on Yoga*, Schoken Books, New York, 1966.

Geeta Iyengar, *Yoga: A Gem for Women*, Timeless Books, New Delhi, 1987.

Judith Lasater, *Relax and Renew*, Rodmell Press, Berkeley, 1995.

Michael Leunig, *A Common Prayer*, Harper Collins, Sydney, 1990.

Silva, Mira and Shyam Mehta, *Yoga the Iyengar Way*, Simon & Schuster, Sydney, 1990.

R.K. Narayan, *Ramayana*, Penguin, 1972.

M. Scott Peck, *The Road Less Travelled*, Touchstone/Simon & Schuster, New York, 1980.

Henry David Thoreau, *Life in the Woods*, Shambhala, 1992.

Upanishads, translated by Eknath Easwaran, Nilgiri Press, 1987.

INDEX

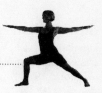

restorative poses, 30–31, 34, 41, 104–10
right-angle stretch, 58, 68
royal yoga, 25

S
salabhasana, 91
salute to the sun, 8, 57, 59, 76–77
samadhi, 19
Sanskrit, 26–27
savasana, 49, 50, 57, 104, 108–10
seasons and cycles, 45–51
sexual continence, 23
side-angle pose, 84–85
sideways extension, 86–87
simhasana, 47
sitting poses, 61–67
slowing down, 127–28
spiritual benefits, 9–13
splits, 57, 98–99
sports' injuries, 4
standing forward bend, 53, 58, 72
standing poses, 50, 53, 57, 59, 78–89, 114, 115
strengthening exercises, 5
stress management, 23
stress reduction, 7, 125–33
stretching, 5
sukhasana, 63
sukhasana twist, 102
supta baddha konasana, 35, 41, 57, 58, 60, 104, 105
supta padangusthasana, 58, 73–75, 119
surya namaskar, 8, 57, 59, 76–77, 118

T
tadasana, 53, 57, 78–79
tailor's pose, 63
tantra, 23
tantra yoga, 25–26
Thoreau, H.D., xv, 125–26
time
   lack of, 37–38
   planning, 128–30
   to practise, 43–44
tiredness or emotional upset, 34–36